I0421155

Empty Your

Fat Bank

By Barry Rabkin

Certified Sports Nutritionist & National
Council on Strength & Fitness Personal Trainer

Please consult your doctor before starting any exercise or nutrition program. We are not liable for any injuries or damages. You train at your own risk.

Dedication

Throughout my chubby youth, my Grandma Irma always worried that I was too heavy. Since I got fit, she always tells me I'm too skinny. Grandma, I love you. This book is proudly dedicated to you.

Table of Contents

#1 Introduction

"Knowing others is intelligence; knowing yourself is true wisdom. Mastering others is strength; mastering yourself is true power."

- Lao-Tzu

Today Is the First Day

Today is your first day on the job as President of your very own bank. This bank was designed and built many years before you were born. This morning you were awarded the keys and combination to the bank vault and complete freedom to run it as you see fit.

As the bank owner, you can withdraw money and spend it on whatever you want. You can also take deposits into your bank vault for safe keeping. Depending on your actions as president, the savings in the bank vault will either grow, or will completely disappear.

But there's one essential twist: You don't store money in your bank. You hold extra energy, also known as calories. When we take in more calories than we use, our bodies store the extra energy as fat, to keep it available for future use.

You've been carrying this bank around with you

your entire life, but no one ever gave you the instruction manual that reveals all the secrets of how it works!

You are reading a comprehensive step-by-step guide on how to empty out your Fat Bank quickly and painlessly with proven strategies that have been effective for thousands of other people just like you.

Big Beginnings

I was obese growing up. Like many others in my situation, I used to stare at myself in the mirror, wishing what I saw would magically change.
I wasn't hoping to look like a supermodel or a profession athlete. I just wanted to look average. I wanted to be able to get a date. I wanted to stop being picked last for team sports. My burning desire was just to be normal.

I kept hoping one day I would look in the mirror and see something different. I felt desperately out of control of my body and certain that I would be stuck that way forever.

When I went off to college, after a few unsuccessful tries I was able to permanently stop smoking. After that, I realized that I might be able to adjust to a healthier lifestyle in other ways too.

I spent the next decade obsessively devouring hundreds of books and thousands of articles and magazines, learning how to take control of my body.

Slowly I went from obese, to average, to athletic. Over the years, I refined my techniques and understanding with endless study and experimentation. I'm now a certified Sport Nutritionist and a National Council on Strength and Fitness Certified Personal Trainer.

All of those endless workouts and late nights of research have been concentrated down into a few basic body transforming principles. You are reading the result of my journey. This is the owner's manual all of our bodies should have come with.

This is the honest, proven, step-by-step guide on how to drop fat and kept it off for the rest of your life. Everyone deserves a body they feel at home in. The Empty Your Fat Bank strategies worked for me and many others just like you. Follow these steps and you'll finally see the body you deserve smiling back at you in the mirror!

Out of Control

Most people feel completely out of control of their weight. They want to lose weight, but, despite their best efforts, they honestly just can't seem to do it. This is not their fault.

People that have raised happy families, run fortune 500 companies, built nations, and created artistic masterpieces still cannot seem to keep their weights in check. It's a problem that affects men and women of every race and every religion in every nation.

We all deserve to look in the mirror and love what we see. After you learn the secrets enclosed in these pages, it will be easy for you to quickly drop fat and keep it off permanently.

The most important thing you can learn about fat loss is this: Your past struggles losing fat have nothing to do with you, and have everything to do with the plan you were following.

On the wrong plan, you will diet and exercise like crazy and see no results at all. No matter how much you workout or starve yourself, the wrong plan will make you gain fat and lose muscle!

I'll teach you how to work with your body, instead of against it, for the results that you want. As you read this book, other people just like you are dropping fat and getting the best bodies of their lives. These people are not harder workers, more committed, smarter or better than you in any way. They are simply following effective Empty Your Fat Bank Secrets.

Effort + Discipline DOES NOT = Fat Loss

Your Fat Loss results are only as good as the plan you're following. I promise you that Following the Empty Your Fat Bank Plan will give you the fastest and easiest fat loss results you've ever experienced in your entire life.

Hopeless & Helpless

If you are like most people you have given up trying to control your body fat. You have probably been taught that to lose fat you need to diet and exercise. But when you do, you get either no results, or a yo-yo effect where your weight drops slightly than shoots up even higher than when you started. This is what leads people to feel helpless and out of control of their body fat.

Even with the best intentions and strictest discipline, it's easy to diet and exercise your way into serious fat gains. The problem is that exercising and dieting can make you gain fat just as easily as they can make you lose it.

To avoid this, you must know and follow a few simple, proven rules. The good news is that, if you follow these rules, you are guaranteed to get the results that you want. You'll also learn how eating **more** and exercising **less** can **lower** your body fat when you follow the Empty Your Fat Bank principals.

Following this plan, you won't need to give up treats, starve yourself, do unhealthy fad diets or spend your life in the gym. The Empty Your Fat Bank strategies will teach you how to effortlessly control your body fat for the rest of your life.

You want control, but you cannot master something

you don't understand. You must take driving lessons and learn the rules of the road before you can use your car, and you must read Empty Your Fat Bank and learn the rules of fat loss before you can master your Fat Bank.

This book teaches a completely new way to think about fat loss, food, and your body. The Fat Bank concept is a truth, an attitude, and for most, a sudden realization.

Think of it like a pair of x-ray glasses that you can put on that will suddenly make things clear and transparent to you. If you don't like what you see, you can take the glasses off and go right back to looking at things as you do today. But for virtually everyone, learning about their Fat Bank gives them new vision that helps them to see how to reach their fitness goals.

Today, the majority of Americans are overweight and over 1/3 are obese. Weight-related diseases are the leading cause of death. The cause of this is very simple: our bodies adapted for millions of years to a food situation that is completely different from modern society.

Your body developed techniques over millions of years of evolution to keep you from starving to death. Your ancestors spent millions of years evolving to survive in a situation where meals were few and far between, and it was starvation, not obesity, that was a leading cause of death.

What Is Food?

If you ask anyone who has trouble keeping their weight down they will tell you: Food is "Evil," Food is "Temptation," Food is "Out to get me," Food is "What's making me fat," Food is "The enemy!" That's understandable. Ask someone drowning what water is and they will tell you it's "Death". But take that drowning person out of the water, and throw him in a scorching dessert with no water, then ask them what water is. They will say it's "Health" "Relief" "Salvation" "Life Itself."

Too much of anything causes problems, even things that we absolutely require to survive. But the problem is not the substance itself, but the excess of it. They key to losing fat is NOT depriving yourself. In fact, as you'll learn, that's the surest road to failure on any weight loss plan.

One common difference you will see between almost all thin people, and all overweight people is how they view food. People that struggle to keep their weight down usually view food as dangerous, sinful, or bad, while people who can control their weight tend to view food as an enjoyable necessity of life, like showers or a good night's sleep. This guide will finally teach you how to use food as a tool to lose fat, rather than as something that makes you fat!

What Is Fat?

Fat is energy. Specifically, fat is stored energy from food. All food has a certain number of calories in it. A big greasy bacon cheeseburger might have 1200 calories, while a big salad with light dressing might have only 300 calories.

Every time you take in more calories from food than your body needs at that time, you store the extra calories as fat. Every extra 3500 calories you eat = 1 pound of added body fat. Likewise, every 3500 calories you burn through living and exercise = 1 pound of body fat lost.

If you're mentally calculating how many treadmill sessions the 20 pounds you want to lose will take you, don't worry about that right now. You didn't put the weight on overnight and you won't lose it overnight. This book does not promise a gimmicky instant fix.

What this teaches is a long term understanding of

food that will change your body and your life forever. This approach will give you a new understanding of food and fat that will make Emptying Your Fat Bank easy and stress free.

Your Body Wants to Be Fat

Why? Because it's better than starving to death! Think of it this way. Most of us use our money to bring us freedom. It helps us do what we want, when we want. In modern society we are used to getting our basic needs met. As long as we hold down a job and don't live outside our means, most of us don't have to worry where our next meal is coming from.

This was not true for most of mankind's history on this planet. Think about how easy it would be for you to lose weight if all you ate were fresh fruits and vegetables. That was the diet of our ancestors, only they weren't grabbing them out of their fridge, they had to take the time and energy to find and gather them in the wild.

Imagine you were living millions of years ago, there are no malls, no cars, no apartments, and no computers. Your primary goal is not to get a new flat screen TV or a bigger house. You just want to survive long enough to find your next meal. There is no processed food, no refrigerators, no vending machines, and no grocery stores. There are no cars. The energy to take you everywhere you go, lift everything you carry, and to do everything you do comes entirely from the calories you eat.

It is almost impossible to get enough calories to fuel your body for basic activities like going hunting for your next meal. Every precious calorie you find means survival. Any extra calories that you consume that are not directly burned for fuel are stored as body fat for later use. Every scrap of fat you can add to your frame buys you a little more time to find food, before starving to death. You can live off fat as a portable energy source even if you can't find food. Fat is survival.

Food is your wealth and your most valuable asset. Body fat is your bank account. It's where you store resources you don't need right now so that you can use them in the future. Foods with a high sugar content give you easily broken down energy, while high calorie foods like fat give you a high density of calories to use and store.

People whose minds and bodies instinctively told them to eat those foods were less likely to starve to death and more likely to pass on their genes. Those genes were eventually passed down to modern man, which is why calorie-dense fatty foods taste, smell, and feel good to us.

Our sweet tooth, love of high carbohydrate, and high fat "comfort foods" have literally been bred into us as a survival instinct over millions of years.

Because calories were such a scarce essential resource for our ancestors, the idea of having too many calories would be just as bizarre as someone today complaining that they have too much money.

If you think about your favorite dishes and popular foods in general, chances are they include a combination of sugar, fat and salt. This is not a coincidence! Our bodies require them in trace quantities and, since they rarely occurred in nature, we're built to store up on them any chance we get.

Today we are still wired to eat all of them we can. Given today's virtually unlimited supply of fat, salt, and sugar everywhere we go, we eat far more than the small amount we need. Eating more of these than we need leads to obesity, hypertension, diabetes, and heart disease.

Your Body Wants to Be

Weak

Why? Because it's better than starving to death!
Muscle is calorically expensive to build and
maintain. Your body is concerned that the energy
cost of supporting the additional muscle will lead
you to starve to death.

It would be like a business hiring employees when it
has no work for them to do. Paying extra money to
workers you don't can lead to bankruptcy. Paying
extra energy to maintain muscle you don't need can
lead to starvation.

You will only grow muscle when you repeatedly
demonstrate to your body that the muscle is needed
and will be used regularly. If you stop using the
muscle, it will slowly shrink since your body wants
to avoid spending unnecessary calories maintaining
calorically expensive muscle that you don't need.
It's like a retail store letting Christmas rush
employees go, when sales slow down after the

holidays.

Your Engine Is Too Fuel Efficient

If gas was $100 a gallon, would you rather be driving an efficient hybrid or a gas-guzzling hummer? If gas was $100, and you had no way of knowing where the nearest gas station was, would you rather have a full tank or an empty one? Your body was designed to use the fuel you gave it efficiently so it could make it to the next fuel source: More food!

To our ancestors, people today complaining about their slow metabolisms, would be like complaining that our cars mileage is **too** good. Your body has evolved over millions of years to be energy efficient so you can survive long periods of starvation.

Unfortunately, the genes that have been bred into us

don't match our modern day needs. Starvation is no longer a serious threat. Instead of being energy efficient, we want to be thinner, stronger, and burn lots of calories so that we can eat whatever we want without storing excess calories as fat.

You want your body to be a gas guzzling sexy Ferrari, while your body wants to be a highly efficient sub-compact hybrid. We are a civilization of sensible 50 mile-per-gallon hybrid Priuses wishing we could be 10 mile-per-gallon Hummers.

The good news is, by applying the secrets in this guide, any hybrid Prius can learn the simple steps to permanently transform themselves into fuel-burning Hummers. You will have the power to control your weight, decide how much fat you want to lose, lose it easily, and keep it off forever.

Your Body Is Suicidal

Our bodies reward us physically and mentally every

time we eat fattening foods. Think of a few of the treats you enjoy most, such as peanut butter, ice cream, burgers, fries, cookies, bacon, chocolate, eggs, cake, pizza and hot dogs. They all taste great, and stimulate serotonin in your brain, the same pleasure chemical that gambling, drugs and sex bring us.

When we are tired or sad, we crave sweets, fats, and carbohydrates, as our body commands us to consume the rich and sugary foods that will make us fat. The excess calories will make us fat, and lead to diseases that will end our lives early. So our bodies are trying to kill us. They are reinforcing behaviors and tempting us to do things that are horrible for our health.

I thought Darwin said we were supposed to be wired to survive, what gives? The truth is, we are living in a situation that we were not designed for. We are fish trying desperately to ride bicycles.

We live in an era in which calories are too abundant instead of too scarce. This has only been true for the past 2,000 years, which is less than .0001% of our species' time on this planet. Given enough time, we will eventually evolve out of our current tastes and instincts toward food.

However, because most overweight people still get a chance to reproduce and pass on their genes before they pass away, this evolutionary change will be extremely slow. Evolution takes hundreds of thousands of years and today we are stuck with our caveman bodies and our caveman survival instincts in our modern fast food world.

How Do You Empty Your Bank Account?

You decide that money is the root of all evil. To walk the path to true enlightenment you must rid yourself of all physical wealth. So you need to empty out your bank account as quickly as possible. You can spend it on anything you want. How would you do it?

There are 3 different possible ways to drain your bank account in a hurry, and for the best, fastest results you should do all 3 at once. You need to minimize the money going into your bank account, and increase your spending both on necessities and recreational luxuries as much as possible.

Minimize Bank Deposits

You deposit as little into your bank account as possible. You would especially want to avoid any particularly large deposits like inheritances, a bonus at work, or taking on extra income from a second job. You might also want to quit your current job, liquidate your investments and shut down anything else that supplies you with an income stream. After all, that incoming money would really slow you down from emptying out your bank account!

Maximize Unnecessary Bank Withdrawals

You increase your spending on necessities as much as possible. You need a roof over your head. You need a car to get to work. You need clothing.

You could meet all those needs by living in a 1 bedroom apartment, leasing a cheap compact car, and shopping at Wal-Mart. But you could fill the same basic needs and spend a lot more in the process. You could get a high-interest mortgage payment on a hotel-sized mansion, buy a Ferrari convertible, and have all your clothing custom tailored by Armani.

No matter what, you have to cover your basic needs to survive. That's going to cost something, but you can control whether covering those needs requires a small amount, or a huge amount of money.

Maximize Unnecessary Fat Bank Withdrawals

You increase your recreational spending on unnecessary products, services and activities as much as possible. There are plenty of things you don't **need**, but that would be fun to buy. You take expensive vacations around the world, get daily Swedish massages, pick up pricey drug habits, buy original Van Gogh paintings, give to charity and build an amusement park in your backyard. Nothing in this group is necessary for survival so theoretically you could spend nothing on recreation at all. Even though you don't **have** to spend anything here, with enough enthusiasm there is virtually no limit to how much you could spend.

Fat Is Not the Enemy

Fat is energy. Fat is survival. Fat is your bodies most fundamental form of wealth. However unlike the primitive lifestyle our bodies spent millions of years adapting to, today we are offered more food than we need. Affordable high calorie food completely surrounds us everywhere we go.

In modern society, most of our Fat Banks are fuller than we would like them to be. Starvation is no longer a serious threat, but our Fat Banks have grown so swollen with excess calories that they have become burdensome to carry with us.

Carrying around our overfilled Fat Banks burdens our joints, slows down our movement, clogs our arteries, and makes us unattractive to potential mates looking for someone fit and healthy. So how do we drain these Fat Banks as quickly as possible? It turns out, the exact same rules apply as emptying out your bank account in real life!

How Do You Empty Your Fat Bank?

There are 3 different possible ways to drain your Fat Bank account in a hurry, and for the best, fastest results you should do all 3 at once. You will need to minimize the calories going into your Fat Bank account, and increase your caloric spending both on necessities and unnecessary activities as much as possible. You deposit into the account by eating and you spend energy from the account by exercising and maintaining your body.

Minimize Fat Bank

Deposits

You deposit as little into your Fat Bank account as possible. In particular you would want to avoid any particularly large deposits like eating an entire chocolate cake or binging on a box of cookies. Those incoming calories would really slow you down from emptying out your Fat Bank account and make it a struggle to use all the caloric energy you have coming in.

Maximize Necessary Fat Bank Withdrawals

You increase your calorie use on necessities as much as possible. You need to supply your muscles and organs with calories to keep them functioning and healthy. You can't do much to change how many calories your organs use, but you can dramatically increase the amount your muscles consume.

The larger your muscles get, the more calories they will require to maintain themselves. With regular strength training you can dramatically increase the amount of muscle you have and increase the calories your body uses maintaining that muscle.

Most bodybuilders and NFL players require 4000-6000 calories per day just to feed their muscles, even if they aren't exercising. No matter what, you have to cover your basic needs to survive, and that's going to cost something, but, by losing or putting on muscle, you can control whether covering those needs requires a small amount or a huge amount of energy.

In medical terms this is known as your BMR or Basal Metabolic Rate. It's the equivalent of the gas your car burns when it's idling in your driveway, without actually going anywhere. Your body requires these calories just to maintain itself while you sit around without any exercise or movement.

You can burn a lot of calories just sitting around, but you can burn even more if you get moving. This brings me to the final way to empty out your Fat Bank.

Maximize Unnecessary Fat Bank Withdrawals

You move around as much as much as possible. There are plenty of things you don't **need** to do, but that would be fun and use up tons of energy. You could run a 10K, take a two hour walk in the park with your dog, help your friend move out of her apartment, take the stairs instead of the elevator, join a pickup basketball game, take an aerobics class, or go out dancing.

Theoretically, you could spend no calories on optional physical activities at all. You don't have to spend anything here, but with enough enthusiasm, there is virtually no limit to how many calories you could burn.

Too Much Money?

At first some will argue, "It's not reasonable to compare having too much money with our ancestors having too much fat. There's nothing bad about having too much money, but having too much fat can kill you." It's not like all fat is bad either, it's only bad if you have too much.

Most people can have at least twenty to forty pounds of extra body fat before they are considered overweight or have any negative health risks associated with their weight. You need a large amount in your Fat Bank before you have any problems from it. But you need to make hundreds of thousands of dollars to be in the highest income tax bracket in America.

Don't you think most people will still think you are crazy if you complain about being in the highest income tax bracket?   You'd still be envied by everyone who was having trouble making ends meet.

The same is true of fat for our ancestors, the "Problem" of excess calories is deeply envied by those suffering from starvation. While one who has too much can simply consume less, it may be difficult or impossible for one who does not have enough to get more.

Your Body Is in Starvation Survival Mode

That means your body wants to use the lowest amount of energy possible and consume the most. Your body fat is your body's bank account and it wants to keep it nice and full. Every time you eat you're making "Fat Bank Deposits" and every time you do physical activity you're making "Fat Bank

Withdrawals."

But there is one other important way your Fat Bank is like a real-life bank. Most people have a spending limit on their bank account as a preventative measure. That means that if a criminal gets your bank card or check book, the criminal can't withdraw your life savings and head over to Mexico to sip Pina Coladas. After that spending limit is reached, the account freezes and the criminal can't take anymore.

The worst that happens is the bank account holder loses $500 (depending on the set limit) and then closes their account when they see the charge, without any permanent harm done. Your body doesn't want you to accidentally empty your Fat Bank account and starve to death, so it has the same type of fail-safe security limits as an actual bank.

Testosterone Is Man's

(And Woman's) Best Friend!

Your body has four primary chemicals that control the rate that your body processes energy and burns fat. The first chemical is called testosterone. Testosterone heats up your fat-burning furnace so huge amounts of fat burn rapidly in a blazing fire. Your testosterone raises your spending limit. It tells your body that's it's okay to get bigger and spend more calories on added muscle and exercise.

Both men and women have testosterone, but men naturally have more of it than women. Most men are already interested in boosting their natural testosterone production, but many women fear increasing their testosterone levels.

Many women assume that, if they increase their testosterone production, they will get enormous muscles, adams apples, deep voices and stylish goatees. Nothing could be further from the truth. Sure, some female body builders look like men, but they have intentionally raised their testosterone to the level of men by using illegal and harmful anabolic steroids.

Women that boost their testosterone naturally using Fat Bank secrets will not become masculine or sprout chest hair. They will be just as feminine, or more feminine than they are today. Just with better curves, more energy, a faster metabolism and less fat!

Naturally increased testosterone levels will result in six important changes for both men and women: lower cortisol levels, reduced fat, more calories burned daily, more muscle tone, higher mental and physical energy levels, and a stronger immune system.

Not a bad deal right? Male or female, if you want to lose fat, testosterone is **the** indispensable secret weapon to quickly empty out your fat vault.

Testosterone gives your Fat Bank the green light for Fat Bank Withdrawals.

Cortisol Kills

Unfortunately you also have cortisol, which gives your Fat Bank the red light for Fat Bank Withdrawals. Cortisol puts your body in a low-energy state where almost no calories are burned. Cortisol slams your Fat Bank vault door shut to prevent fat from leaving.

Your body produces cortisol in stressful situations when it panics and thinks you are at risk of starving. Cortisol puts your body into a hibernation state which locks your Fat Bank down to stop any more calories from leaving the vault. This cortisol survival mechanism is hardwired into all of our bodies to make our fat stores last until we can find more food.

The low-energy state that cortisol puts you in doesn't just make it difficult to lose fat. High cortisol levels **does** increase our fat storage, especially increased abdominal fat, but that's just the tip of the iceberg.

Cortisol makes our body use less energy by reducing our mental and physical systems to low power mode. Because cortisol focuses your body's systems on using the least energy possible, your body doesn't operate nearly as well as it could at full power.

High cortisol levels have been proven to impair your learning, memory, and decision-making abilities. Cortisol weakens your immune system so you get sicker, more often and take longer to recover. Cortisol has been linked to blood sugar imbalances like hyperglycemia, diabetes, and higher blood pressure. Cortisol leads to decreased bone density, decreased muscle tissue, and increased risk of both heart disease and strokes.

Put quite simply, "Cortisol Kills!" So how do we

stop our bodies from producing this deadly toxin? The good news is there are 4 very specific things that lead to cortisol production, all of which can be easily avoided if you know the Fat Bank secrets. The next section provides you with a complete road map to lead you to an Empty Fat Bank and a cortisol free body.

How to Close Your Fat Bank Vault: Cortisol and You

There are four specific trip wires that will make your body produce cortisol if you hit them. Each of these trip wires put your metabolism into a deep freeze and stop you from effectively removing calories from your Fat Bank. Despite your best effort to empty out your Fat Bank, if you walk into any of these trip wires, your Fat Bank vault will slam shut and make it virtually impossible to lose fat.

These trip wires are permanent in each of us, and there is no way to disarm them. But, if you know where the trip wires are and what triggers them, you can easily watch for them and avoid them. Just step around them and leave your Fat Bank permanently open for withdrawals. This guide shows you exactly where the cortisol trip wires are so that you can easily step over them without setting them off.

Why do we have these trip wires? Each trip wire tells our body that it is being threatened and may no longer have a reliable food source. This switches your body into emergency mode and puts your system into a peak efficiency, low energy stasis mode so that it can use the least energy possible to guarantee that its limited available energy stores (fat) will last long enough to make it to the next energy source (food) before you starve to death.

People that didn't produce cortisol used lots of energy, even when there was no food around (they were Hummers when gas stations were few and far between), and they ran out of gas (fat) before they could make it to the next station. They died before they could pass their genes on, so the genes were slowly weeded out of our civilization.

People that produced more cortisol survived (they were sub-compact hybrid cars when gas stations were few and far between), so they could make it long enough to get to the next fuel source. This efficiency kept them alive and healthy, which made them more attractive mates, and, because their genes were desirable, they were passed on, all the way down to you and me.

#2 Food & You:

How to Make Deposits into Your Fat Bank

"You better cut the pizza in four pieces because I'm not hungry enough to eat six." - Yogi Berra

"Statistics show that of those who contract the habit of eating, very few survive." - George Bernard Shaw

Crazy or Cautious?

Your body is scared that you're going to starve to death. It seems crazy until you remember that your ancestors spent their entire lives just trying to get enough food to ward off starvation. Your body is always ready to switch to starvation survival mode when it puts all its systems on low power to ensure you can survive long enough to make it to your next meal.

This is why starvation diets don't work—your system goes into a cortisol-induced stasis. Your Fat Bank vault door slams shut, so you virtually stop burning calories. When you do eat again, you immediately gain the fat back and then some!

When your body is starved and your cortisol is high, your body cannibalizes your muscle both for energy and to get rid of the muscle that is using up calories that your body is trying to conserve. That muscle was constantly burning calories to maintain itself, so, when the muscle is gone (even if you're eating the same as you always did), your body now needs less calories.

The calories that your muscle **had** been burning is now going unused and is stored as fat! This is the single biggest reason that the diet industry is a multi-billion dollar market in which people spend decades trapped, bouncing from one miracle product to another, dropping and gaining weight in endless yo-yo diets.

With crash and fad diets, most of the weight you lose is muscle. Because your muscles had been burning calories, when when you do go back to eating normally, you not only gain your initial weight back, everything your muscles would be burning gets gained as fat too! Scary stuff, but don't worry. Keep reading, I'll teach you how to prevent this from happening!

Cut Your Expenses and Put the Savings in Your Fat Bank Account

Let's go back to the Fat Bank analogy. Let's say you are single and make $40,000 a year. With taxes, rent, car payments, utilities, groceries, entertainment, and vacations at the end of each year, you seem to break even. You can pay for all your expenses, but you have nothing left to show for it—your money coming in matches your money going out.

One day your boss informs you that your company is going through hard times and has to cut your pay to make ends meet. This year you will only be making $30,000, but you still need to make sure you can cover all your expenses. You know money will be tight.

You prepare by downsizing to a cheaper apartment

and switching to a car with lower monthly payments. You make ends meet, and, at the end of the year, you can pay off all your bills, but you have no savings left over. Again, your income matches your expenses.

You earned less than last year, but you still were able to pay all your expenses by adjusting to lower expenses that your lower income could cover. At the end of that year, things in your industry have turned around. Your boss is again able to pay you your standard $40,000 annual salary.

Last year, that salary wasn't enough to leave you any savings at the end of the year, but this year you downsized to cheaper more efficient circumstances. With your current rent and car you only need $30,000 to cover everything. At the end of the year, you are left with $10,000 extra dollars, which you deposit into your bank account as savings.

Want to Be Fat? Starve Yourself!

Many people who get frustrated trying to control their weight try fasting, starvation diets, skipping meals, and in essence trying to go "cold turkey" on food, as if they were quitting smoking or drugs. The difference is, unlike nicotine, no body can survive without food.

Your body reacts very badly to being starved. Your cortisol shoots through the roof, which not only slows your metabolism down, but also decreases your muscle tissue which slows your calorie-burning furnace for the future. You may look down at the scale and see that you've lost weight, when really, you've only lost calorie burning muscle!

Even if you are only eating the same amount as before your diet, now with less muscle you will gain more fat. Losing muscle that had been burning calories, leaves you with extra energy that gets saved in your Fat Bank. Starvation dieting is like using a wrecking ball to remove a door knob, or a machete to cut a hang nail. You're not just going to lose the problem area, you're going to damage things you wanted to keep too!

Want to Lose Weight? Gain Weight!

When you look fit, people ask if you've lost weight. This is because almost no one understands the most fundamental truth of fat loss. It's not weight that's the problem! It's fat that is the problem. Weight can be your friend. Weight in the form of calorie burning muscle is the solution to getting rid of weight in the form of fat.

Maintaining and gaining muscle is the most important long-term change you can make to keep your fat down. If you're losing fat, gaining muscle, and maintaining your overall weight, you are completely transforming your body, but it will never show up on the scale. A six foot tall man man who weighs two hundred and thirty pounds could be extremely lean and muscular, or fat and out of shape. The weight itself does not tell us the whole story. The more muscle you put on, the **easier** it will be to keep your fat down since muscle burns tons of calories.

Weight in the form of muscle is one of the best tools you have to eliminate fat for good. The question is not, have you lost weight? The question is, have you lost fat?

Your Body Only Understands One Thing: Food

Let's say you skip breakfast because you're in a hurry. Now you know that you're grabbing a burger and fries with your friends for lunch and you won't starve, but there is no way to explain this to your body.

Your body is busy with its "Caveman Concerns" that you won't be able to spear a bison on the hunt and will go hungry. Your body is worried it will starve, so it spikes up your cortisol levels to slow your system down and burn less calories.

If you convince your body that you're not going to starve, it won't produce cortisol. There's no way to rid your body of these "Cavemen Concerns," but you can speak in the one language it understands. Food! If you go too long without eating (three to four hours) your cortisol levels start to rise.

You don't need to eat Thanksgiving dinner-sized feasts every 4 hours to keep your metabolism up. All you need is a small snack to convince your system that it's not starving and that there's no need to panic. The more calories you eat, the lower your cortisol levels drop and the more calories you burn.

Any small meal will drop your cortisol down and rev your metabolism back up. If you skip meals, your body produces cortisol and slams the brakes on your metabolism. Your energy levels and mental alertness will decrease and your testosterone and growth hormone levels will drop off.

Your body doesn't know if or when it's next meal will be. The last thing your body would want to do is waste precious calories building or maintaining calorically-expensive muscle, so the testosterone that encourages its growth has to go!

There are hundreds of myths and misunderstandings about diet and nutrition, but the single most common and most damaging myth is that skipping breakfast and meals in general helps you lose fat. Nothing could be further from the truth. When you are in a starvation induced cortisol bath, most of the weight you lose will be muscle, not fat. To avoid this, eat small healthy meals every three to four hours.

Avoid Liquid Diets

I've had friends who would routinely drink a six pack of soda every single day. It's no surprise that all that sugar made it hard to keep their weight down. Except for water and tea, most drinks are chocked full of sugar and calories that will sabotage your fat loss efforts.

Sports drinks, soda, and energy drinks all put tons of extra calories in your system. Most beverages are processed with a ton of added sugar and all fiber removed, so they don't ultimately satisfy you. Stick to water, skim milk, and tea when you're thirsty and stop drinking your calories other than for pre-workout energy boosts or post-workout protein shakes. The sugar you eat before and after your workout is rapidly used, so, as long as you do it at the right time, you can indulge in your favorite treats and still lose fat.

Ectomesoendo

Our genes give our bodies instructions to develop in different ways. Some of us are naturally taller where others are shorter. Just like we have different color eyes, hair, and skin based on our genes, they also help determine our physical shape. There are three different body types:

Some of us can eat anything and everything in sight and still stay rail thin. These people have an Ectomorph body type. Ectomorphs are naturally skinny and have an easy time keeping fat off, but have a harder time putting on muscle than other body types. Ectomorphs have a marathon runners build. Celebrity examples of this body type include Gwyneth Paltrow and Brad Pitt.

Some people gain weight if they even look at a dessert, but are naturally more muscular than Ectomorphs. These people have an Endomorph body type. Endomorphs are naturally more muscular, with bigger bones and higher levels of body fat. Endomorphs have an easy time putting on muscle, but a harder time staying slim. Endomorphs have a football line backer's build. Celebrity examples of this body type include Jennifer Lopez, Seth Rogen and John Candy.

Some people seem to build muscle just by lifting their TV remote. These people have a Mesomorph body type. Mesomorphs are a blend of the other two body types with thicker bones, less body fat, and more muscle. Mesomorphs have a body builder's or sprinter's build. Celebrity examples of this body type include Jessica Biel, Ron Coleman, and LL Cool J.

The Power Is Yours

You can't change your skin color or your eye color. If you've finished puberty and stopped growing, you can't get any taller. But regardless of your genetic body type, you can make very fast progress transforming your body. You will see the fastest results by working with your body type rather then against it.

If an Ectomorph diets and exercises, they will shed fat incredibly quickly. Gaining muscle for an Ectomorph is a little tougher. They'll need to eat lots and cut down on cardio, so all of the energy that they are putting in their system can go straight to muscular development.

Endomorphs will have an easy time putting on muscle and gaining strength. If an Endomorph wants to lose weight, they will need to emphasize portion control, and get plenty of exercise. Mesomorphs also have an easy time putting on muscle, but they still have to exert some portion control to stay skinny.

Beginner and intermediate strength trainers will experience fast fat loss and strength gain results simultaneously if they diet, workout, and exercise.

For Advanced strength trainers or "Hard Gainers" (People who have a difficult time gaining muscle) results will come faster if they focus completely on fat loss or muscle gain at any one time.

First, they will go through a "Bulking Phase" in which they will exercise less, emphasize strength training and eat everything in sight to add muscle and fat. Following this they enter a "Cutting" or "Shedding Phase" in which they will eat less and focus on exercising.

They will only strength train often enough to maintain their new muscle and will primarily focus on diet and exercise to shed the fat that they put on in their bulking phase.

No matter what phase you are in, what's on your plate today will be on your body tomorrow.

Slow Metabolism? Eat More!

It's morning and you slam your alarm clock off and slowly crawl out of bed, semi-conscious, feeling weak, uncoordinated and unaware. Some of this is because you're still tired, but the main culprit is your high level of cortisol. You have fasted for 8-12 hours since your last meal. Your cortisol levels are through the roof and your testosterone and growth hormone have hit rock bottom.

If you skip breakfast, your just continuing this situation throughout your entire day, letting your cortisol levels rise higher and higher, and your metabolism getting slower and slower until it's barely functioning at all. The first thing you have to do to reverse this is to "break the fast" with breakfast! Eat and not only will you knock your cortisol levels down and raise your testosterone back up, you'll feel more awake and more energetic.

How often have you heard somebody complain that they have a slow metabolism? Maybe you've spent time with them and noticed that, just like they say, they only eat a small amount, but they **still** gain weight.

Assuming they don't have a rare thyroid problem throwing off their hormones, the most common cause of their slow metabolism is skipping breakfast or going a long time between meals so their cortisol levels spike up and their metabolism slows down to a crawl.

So what can you do to keep your cortisol levels as low as possible? Your body processes foods high in sugar faster than anything else, and the minute it finishes processing it, your cortisol levels start creeping up again. If you eat more whole grains, fruits, vegetables, lean proteins, and fiber, they are all slowly broken down, keeping your cortisol levels low and your testosterone high for much longer.

Slow Down!

Most of us are in such a rush that we practically inhale our meals. Instead of slowly chewing, pausing to savor every bite, we just throw the food down our throats. Not only does eating this way leave us feeling unsatisfied, we also tend to overeat.

It takes about 20 minutes from the time we eat food for it to reach our stomach and to register to our brain. If you wolf down your food until you feel full, your brain is only registering what you ate 20 minutes ago, and you are likely to feel uncomfortably overstuffed after the meal, when the rest of the food finally hits your stomach.

It's common after overeating to feel sluggish, overstuffed, and like you need a nap. This feeling comes from all the blood in our body flowing to our stomachs to try to digest the mountain of food. This leaves the rest of our body feeling de-energized. This tiredness often leads people to have after meal sweets, cigarettes, or coffee, which serve as pick-me ups at the time but cause an even worse crash later.

So how do we break the cycle? How do we slow down and actually feel good and energized after we finish eating? Make conversation. Don't talk with your mouth full. Chew your food slowly. Drink plenty of water before and during your meal. Not only will you enjoy your food more, and feel more energized after you eat, you'll lose fat too!

6 Packs Won't Give You a 6 Pack

"Once, during Prohibition, I was forced to live for days on nothing but food and water." - W. C. Fields

Drinking alcohol in moderation has medically proven health benefits. If you enjoy drinking, there's no need to stop. You can have an occasional drink and still dramatically change your body. While drinking in moderation is absolutely fine, having more than a drink or two a day will seriously hinder your fat loss efforts.

Alcohol reduces your metabolism because it is a depressant and will severely weaken you for your workout if you try to drink before. Alcohol also slows down your protein processing, screws with your sleep patterns, and lowers your testosterone, all of which make it hard to get the best results from your workouts. Most alcoholic drinks have a fair number of calories. I've known people that lost 10 pounds in a month, simply by cutting out alcoholic beverages for 30 days. Drinking in moderation will not get in the way of your fat loss goals. But, if you drink regularly and want to lose fat, cut back on booze and start relying on your workouts for a healthier way to relax and relieve stress.

Bigger Is Not Better

You build and repair muscle after workouts by supplying them with protein. After a certain point, larger amounts of protein in a meal will not lead to faster muscle gains because your body can only absorb 25-45 grams of protein per sitting. That's the amount in two medium pork chops or a large chicken breast. Anything you eat above that range cannot be used, and will just be stored as fat.

Most protein powder supplements recommend you consume 60-100 grams of protein before and after your workout. They do this simply in the hopes of selling you more of their protein, not to increase your strength or muscle mass. If you are strength training and want to increase your protein intake, space it out evenly over the day, don't try to get your day's supply of protein in a single meal. Consuming 6 chicken breasts or 3 protein shakes will not make you strong, it will only make you store the extra calories as fat. Stay within 25-45 grams of protein per meal and they will go to build your muscles, not your waistline.

The Domino Effect

When you roll a tiny snowball down a hill, it picks up more snow and grows as it rolls. What started as a harmless pebble-sized snow clump at the top of the hill becomes a massive frost boulder capable of serious damage by the time it reaches the bottom of the slope.

Eating is the same way. We all have certain foods and beverages that are difficult for us to eat in moderation. For these items, the first bite or sip may be harmless, but it becomes the snowball that we toss down the hill. By the base of the mountain, it's an enormous calorie laden wrecking ball soaring toward our waistlines. If you've ever opened up a new bag of chips while watching television and been shocked to look down later and find the bag empty, you know what I'm talking about.

Consider these items dominos: The first domino falling isn't significant by itself, but that first domino's fall starts a chain reaction that makes **all** the dominos fall. Your domino foods and beverages are likely to be different than mine, but it's important to know the enemy so that you can avoid them. Next time a bite or a sip turns into many more take note of what you've been consuming. Sugary treats, chips, alcohol, and caffeine are particularly common domino foods and drinks since they cause your system to spike and then rapidly crash, leaving you craving more to pick yourself back up.

Your domino foods may not be particularly unhealthy, but you should still avoid them when you're trying to lose fat. Dried fruit is a domino food for me. Orange juice is a domino for my friend John. Both are high in electrolytes and vitamins, and neither are inherently unhealthy. But, the problem is that it's almost impossible for us to have them in moderation. That first serving automatically leads to 10 more.

I would recommend avoiding domino foods and beverages entirely when you're trying to lose fat. Don't buy them—they can only sabotage your efforts. If you have them in your house, give them to friends or box them up and put them somewhere you won't see them.

If you want to consume domino items, don't make a meal out of them, just have a bite or a sip for taste. If you're sitting next to the serving dish, it's easy to unconsciously go back for seconds and thirds without even realizing it. Take a small serving onto your plate and put the serving dish away. If you're at a party, leave the area that the serving dish is in. Focus on chewing slowly and fully experiencing every single bite. If you take more than one serving, work out afterward to use up all the calories you just put in your system.

Want to Lose Fat? Eat Fat!

It would be easy for someone to think, "Fat is high in calories. I should completely cut fat from my diet to help me lose weight." The problem is that your body actually needs fat to function. Testosterone is made from fat, and testosterone is the chemical that keeps your metabolism high, keeps your muscles growing, and your cortisol levels low.

So, while going on a low fat diet is a smart strategy to help you control your calories, you don't want to reduce your fat intake to below 10% of your total calories. If you cut your cut intake under that, your body will stop producing testosterone and your cortisol will skyrocket, slowing your fat loss gains to a crawl.

Snake Venom Is Organic!

Most people think organic and natural foods are good for them. That is completely untrue. While some organic and natural foods are healthy, most are just as high in fat and sugar as their processed, non-organic versions. It is easy to gain a huge amount of fat, even while eating a purely organic diet. Whether organic or not, almost all breakfast cereals, peanut butter, apple sauce, fruit juices, nuts, and canned fruits are extremely high in fat and/or sugar. Organic does not mean it's good for you or that it will help you empty your Fat Bank. Remember, drinking olive oil (100% pure fat) is all natural. In fact, eating arsenic is organic. That doesn't mean it's good for your body!

If you're buying organic food and assuming it's

good for you, you're probably getting much more fat and sugar in your diet than you realize. Get in the habit of checking the nutritional facts and making sure that what you're putting in your body is not just organic, but also low in fat, salt and sugar.

Cheat Your Way to a Better Body!

So what's the point of dieting if it means you have to give up all the foods that you live for? What if you could lose fat while eating the sweets and treats you love? It's counter-intuitive but the truth is, cheating on your diet can be the best thing for your fat loss. Not only do your indulgences make it easier to stay on the diet, they can even **increase** your fat loss results. Empty Your Fat Bank strategies will minimize your cortisol, even while you diet and exercise. But your cortisol levels will still creep up slightly after a full week of serious fat loss.

The good news is that you can have a lot of fun knocking your cortisol levels back down flat. As long as you've been exercising and eating healthy, you should feel free to reward your hard work with one indulgence meal every week. Hit a Chinese buffet, get that second slice of ice cream cake at your friend's birthday or wolf down pizza and wings while you watch the game.

Just follow 2 rules and your tasty treats will kill your cortisol, grow your muscles, and speed up your metabolism.

#1 Get in a savage strength training session before you eat. Focus on major muscle groups like your chest, back, and legs that generate lots of force and use lots of energy. Get some carbohydrates in your system before the session so you can really push yourself the whole time. Aim to exercise for 30-60 intense minutes.

This exercise session will create a severe energy debt

in your muscles. The calories from your cheat day will replenish this energy debt in your muscles, and you won't gain an ounce of fat. This is also the best way to get serious results from strength training, even while dieting. The nutrients and protein from your food will go straight to your hungry muscles and help them get bigger and stronger.

#2 Front load your meals. You can rev up your metabolism with a massive meal in the morning or afternoon, and you will have all day to use the calories. If you eat late at night and then sleep, the energy you've supplied your body with will go unused and will be stored as fat. So, make sure you have at least 4-8 hours after the feast before you go to sleep. This extra time gives your body an opportunity to burn the calories instead of storing them as fat.

Stealth Fat

The problem that most overweight people struggle with is **not** a lack of discipline or difficulty avoiding indulgences they know they shouldn't eat. What's making them fat is the foods they eat that they don't realize are bad for them. These hidden threats are what make people feel out of control and powerless to change their bodies. If you feel like you're eating healthy and still gaining fat, it's easy to feel helpless. But, the truth is that you are in complete control of what you put into your body. You just need to know the foods that are sabotaging your fat loss efforts, so you don't inadvertently ruin your diet without even knowing it!

You know that high fructose corn syrup is one of the leading causes of obesity in the USA. High fructose syrup increases the production of ghrelin (the hormone that your stomach releases that makes you feel hunger) and stops the production of leptin (the hormone that makes you feel satisfied from a meal). You know that high fructose corn syrup is sneaked into the vast majority of processed foods.

You also know that high fructose corn syrup is also called fructose, fructose syrup, or corn syrup on most nutrition facts labels to try to hide what it really is from consumers. So, you check for corn syrup on labels and avoid products that contain it.

The increased use of high fructose corn syrup in the American food industry corresponds perfectly with the American rise of obesity. Even though high fructose corn syrup isn't listed on the side of product labels as fat, your body will almost immediately store it as fat. While fruits and vegetables are slowly broken down by your system, and even sugar can be used by every part of your body, corn syrup can only be broken down by your liver. If you give your body more high fructose syrup than your liver can use at that time (which is an incredibly tiny amount), all the rest gets stored as fat. Unlike fruits, vegetables, whole grains, lean proteins, and fat, high fructose corn syrup doesn't make your body release the hormone leptin which makes you feel satisfied from your meal. Because high fructose corn syrup won't make you feel full unlike natural foods, you'll eat larger quantities of it and still feel unsatisfied and want more.

Fat's Arch-Nemesis

Fortunately, there is an "Anti-High Fructose Corn Syrup" High fructose corn syrup is the comic book arch-villain and this miraculous substance is the super hero! Unlike corn syrup, this makes you feel full for a long time, isn't stored as fat and doesn't have any calories. It's all natural, affordable, easy to find, and healthy for everyone. It's called fiber, and it's one of your best tools to help you lose fat.

Fiber is in virtually all fruits, vegetables, and whole grains. Fiber has no calories, and will not be stored as fat. Your stomach breaks fiber down very slowly so you feel fuller longer. Cut high fructose corn syrup from your diet and replace it with more fiber. Even if you're eating less than you're used to, instead of feeling hungry and deprived, your meals will leave you more satisfied than ever.

#3 Exercise & You:

How to Make Withdrawals from Your Fat Bank

"Perfection is achieved perfection not when there is nothing left to add, but when there is nothing left to take away." – Antoine de Saint-Exupery

"It is exercise alone that supports the spirits, and keeps the mind in vigor." - Cicero

H.I.T. Me!

Are you ready for the 2 most common fitness myth out there? I guarantee you've heard someone say, "I'd like to get in shape, but I just don't have time to spend my whole life in the gym!" In truth, you don't have to! Short intense workouts make the best use of your time, increase your testosterone, keep your cortisol levels low, and get you out of the gym and back to living your life.

High Intensity Interval Training (HIIT), TABATA Intervals and Supersets are the best ways to quickly burn fat and gain muscle. With 20-60 minute workouts 3-4 times a week you'll see dramatic results.

It's proven that after an hour of intense exercise your testosterone drops like a rock. So you're not only wasting your time, but your draining the system that give you fast results from your training. The best way to get fast results is not by spending every waking moment working out, but simply by doing quick intense sessions that keep your testosterone levels maxed out.

Inactive Lifestyle=Fast Results!

How about this common complaint? "I want to get in shape, but I have to spend all day sitting around my school or office!" Good news! That's the ideal climate for fast gains from your workouts.

When your body has many demands on it, it's recovery systems are overtaxed and gains come slowly. If you spend most of your time resting and recovering, your body can make the fastest possible gains from strength training and intense exercise.

Being inactive at your job or school is not an excuse for excess body fat. The more you can rest between workouts, the faster you will make progress. The lack of movement at your job or school isn't what's holding you back from fat loss.

That rest is an ideal opportunity to fully recover from workouts and improve your body. The lack of exercise done **outside** work or school is what's keeping you from taking advantage of the prime recovery time.

Kill Your Gym

Many people hate gyms. They hate taking the time to commute and change clothes, paying the membership fees, waiting in line for the equipment, paying a personal trainer $80 an hour or trying to figure out the complicated equipment while everyone else in the gym watches and passes judgement. If this describes you, don't worry.

You absolutely **do not** need to join a gym to get in

the best shape of your life. You only need your body and a knowledge of basic bodyweight exercises.

 Learning these techniques transforms fitness from an external, costly inconvenience into a free, convenient lifetime skill. Strength and fat loss will no longer be something you pay personal trainers, gyms, and exercise equipment manufacturers for. Strength and exercise becomes something you take with you wherever you go.

All that your muscles understand is work. Whether you lift metal weights, or your own body weight, your muscles can't tell the difference. With my techniques, you can change your body's leverage to make your body weight very easy to lift or very challenging.

Learn basic bodyweight exercises like pushups, lunges, squats, pullups, and situps. Skip the gym membership and expensive equipment and cut straight to a lifetime of free muscle gain and weight loss!

Less Is More

I'm in the best shape of my life, and I exercise for a half hour a day two to four days a week. That's ninety to one hundred and twenty minutes a week, the length of one movie. It's enough time to lose one or two pounds of fat a week and gain serious muscle!

The benefits of these workouts goes beyond physical changes. These workouts energize and de-stress me, and are easily the most important thing I do every week to keep myself at my best. You never have to feel guilty about taking the time away from your family, friends, or work to exercise. The little time these workouts take gives you dramatically more energy and focus to bring to every moment of the rest of your life. Friends and family will often want to join you, so you can spend time together even while you enjoy the benefits of exercise.

Making exercise a part of your life doesn't have to take much time and there's actually a lot of evidence that spending too much time exercising will actually hurt your fat loss efforts. Countless clinical research studies have shown that cortisol steadily rises from the physical stress of intense exercise after thirty-sixty minutes of exercise.

The time range depends on the intensity of the exercise. While an athlete could walk for an hour without any strain, after thirty minutes of power lifting or sprints, anyone's system will be overloaded.

When you put too much physical stress on your body, your body goes into high alert and starts hysterically trying to protect itself. Your body thinks: "You're burning too many calories too fast. I'm going to lose my fat stores, starve, and die!" So, your body drops anchor and starts spewing out cortisol to slow your system down and lower your testosterone.

If you think of your fat as an energy bank, it's trying to slam the vault door shut so that you can't take out any more precious calories. Since testosterone helps you build muscle and burn fat, this is the exact opposite of what you want to happen in terms of adding muscle, increasing your metabolism, and burning fat.

So where did the myth that you need to spend your life in the gym come from? Plenty of steroid and growth hormone fueled body builders will lift weights for three to four hours every day and describe their fitness routine in interviews. Their bodies can handle these workouts for one simple reason. They are injecting drugs that artificially raise their testosterone, regardless of how much cortisol is in their systems.

Steroid users can raise their testosterone levels to 20 times the level of non-users. The cortisol produced from these endless workouts gets overpowered by their steroids-raised testosterone levels, so they continue to burn fat and build muscle.

Despite the short-term results, steroids are not a recommended fitness tactic for three reasons: Steroids are illegal, they make your bodies natural testosterone production shut down, and finally, they are linked to a wide variety of physical disorders including, liver failure, depression and heart disease.

So, for the non-drug user, long workouts will do

more harm than good. So how can you burn plenty of calories exercising and still keep your cortisol levels low? Keep your workouts short and intense so that your cortisol levels stay low and your testosterone levels stay high. Less time working out means faster results.

Increase Your Energy!

If you feel like you never have any energy for your workouts, let me share some effective secrets to max out your energy levels for every workout. The most common cause of low energy for workouts is low blood sugar, so try to eat at least two meals before your workout. Don't exercise or strength train on an empty stomach.

If you get cramps from eating, drink some juice, milk, or a sports drink so that you have some fast fuel for your system. Drink plenty of water both during exercise and throughout the day so that you don't get dehydrated.

If you want to workout twice in one day, try to time the exercise sessions at least six hours and two meals apart to get your energy back up. Keep your workout between thirty to sixty minutes to keep your cortisol levels low and your testosterone levels high.

Before you begin demanding exercise, warm up your system for five to ten minutes with light cardio until you break a sweat, and then do easy warm up sets before doing intense strength training.

If you want to exercise for more than 30 minutes, limit caffeine and stimulant supplements before your workout. Caffeine is an effective tool to temporarily increase your energy levels, but the increase is followed by a crash soon after. If you're doing challenging strength training or sprints, give yourself at least one or two minutes between sets to give your central nervous system a chance to refresh for the next set.

Get at least eight hours of sleep the night before. Everyone's energy levels are highest at a different point of the day depending on their biological clock. Some people are freshest in the morning, others are freshest in the afternoon or evening. Try to schedule your workouts to coincide with your peak energy time. If that is unrealistic given your schedule, you're still better off working out a non-peak time, rather than not working out at all. The best workout schedule is the one you will stick to.

Want to Be Thin? Gain Weight!

Weight is your friend. Weight is, ironically, the best long-term tool you have for weight loss. Every pound on your body requires about fifteen calories a day to maintain itself, even if you don't exercise and just lay around. The calories your body uses this way is called your Basal Metabolic Index.

Let's assume you've been consuming two thousand calories a day before you started dieting. You lose a combination of fat and muscle and your weight drops. You go back to eating the same two thousand calories as before. But you don't just gain back the fat you lost. You get fatter!

This happens because muscle burns more calories than fat. This is the leading cause of a multi-billion dollar fad diet industry that doesn't work. Fat loss must be your goal, not weight loss. There are several important changes you must make to your training plan if you want to lose fat, instead of just lose weight.

Focus on strength training, not just cardio. This will maintain and strengthen your muscles so they help you lose fat and keep it off for good. Your diet must support muscular growth, not just weight loss. You should always eat or drink something before you workout so you have the energy to challenge your muscles and encourage them to grow.

You also need to eat plenty of protein to fuel your muscle growth and recovery. Focus on lean proteins, such as non-fried chicken or fish, rather than high fat proteins like peanut butter, bologna, hot dogs, or hamburgers.

Throw Out Your Scale!

Body weight is not the problem. Body Fat is the problem. No one is overweight, we are "overfat." It is a very important distinction that completely changes how you measure progress and your long-term results. Throw out your scale. Measure your progress using pictures, BMI, increased strength and calipers, not just your scale.

The best way to control your weight long term is by gaining muscle that will burn calories all day even when you're not exercising. Instead of focusing on what the scale says, chart your progress by how you actually look in the mirror, your body fat percentage, and your overall strength increases.

If your weight stays the same but you've gained muscle and lost fat, you have to look beyond the scale to see any progress. If you lose 10 pounds and it's all muscle, you're worse off than if you hadn't lost an ounce! All losing 10 pounds of muscle does is lower your metabolism, guaranteeing future fat gains and making you weaker!

Whatever your current weight is, let's imagine you wake up tomorrow and you've magically lost 10 pounds of fat and gained 10 pounds of muscle. Do you think you're going to look different in the mirror? Do you think you're going to look better walking along the beach in your swim suit? Do you think you're going to feel stronger and more energetic? Yes, yes and yes!

But the scale won't notice any difference at all. Who

cares if your weight loss is zero, if you look like a hero? So forget about weight loss because the scale can't tell you if you're making progress towards your goals! If you lose 10 pounds and it's all muscle than you're just guaranteeing future fat gains! Focus on pictures, strength gains, and body fat calipers as your tools to measure what really matters and to reach your real goal: fat loss!

Muscle Never Turns to Fat

There is a common myth that muscle will turn into fat over time. It is completely untrue, but the misconception comes from something we've all seen. Many ex-jocks put on a ton of weight after they stop playing sports.

They don't gain fat because their muscles turn into fat. They gain fat because they keep eating the same way that they used to when they exercised, but they stop using that energy by exercising. As a result, every calorie they don't use gets stored as fat.

If you were eating 5000 calories a day and using 5000 calories to fuel your body and exercise, then you won't gain an ounce. If you stop using up all those calories exercising but keep eating 5000 calories a day, suddenly everything you had been burning through exercise now gets stored as fat! Ex-athletes' muscle mass actually slows their fat gains by keeping their metabolism high, but not as high as when they had the muscle and were exercising.

Over time, if they don't use their muscles at all, their bodies will assume their muscles are no longer needed. Their muscles will atrophy and their metabolism will decrease. If an ex-athlete works out their muscles once a week they can maintain their muscle and high metabolism indefinitely.

Muscle and fat are two completely different tissues and one cannot transform into the other. Just like you can't turn lead into gold, muscle will never turn into fat. More muscle will **always** help you avoid gaining fat by burning calories that would otherwise be stored as fat.

Don't Hit the Road with an Empty Gas Tank

Many people have heard rumors that we burn a higher percentage of fat when we exercise on an empty stomach. Without any other fuel sources to work off, our bodies digest our fat tissue for energy. If you put food in your system, your body will use that food for energy during exercise, instead of running purely off of fat. This rumor is absolutely true, but it only tells you half of the story.

While your muscles can use fat to survive, glucose (sugars from processed foods) make a **much** better fuel source. It's the difference between starting a fire with wet matches versus starting a fire with jet fuel and a blow torch! Because of the fast energy glucose gives your muscles, you will be able to exercise much more intensely and push your body harder.

This more intense a workout is, the more calories you can burn! Compared to working out on an empty stomach, a smaller percentage of those burned calories will come from fat, but you will still burn more calories overall.

Put another way, it's not enough to have a high percentage, you want a high **total** amount. Would you rather I give you 100% of $1, or 50% of $100? The first will leave you with $1, while the 2nd will leave you with $50. You want a higher **total** amount, not a higher percentage. So, always fill up your gas tank before you hit the road.

A smaller percentage of the calories you burn will come from fat, but you will be able to exercise so much more intensely that a higher **total** number calories will come from fat. Light exercise will only burn calories while the exercise is being performed.

Doing any exercise intensely burns fat during the workout and creates an energy debt that burns calories throughout the day, which is called "Excess Post Exercise Oxygen Consumption" or EPOC. This "Afterburn" keeps you burning more calories even 24-72 hours **after** your workout is completed!

You Are a Cannibal!

When you workout on an empty stomach, fat isn't the only thing that your body breaks down for fuel. Your body also breaks down your muscle for energy. Your muscle gets left alone, if you provide it food to use as fuel instead.

If you want to burn more calories, burn more fat, and leave your hard earned muscle intact, get a snack, meal, juice, sports drink, or shake before you workout. Your body cannibalizes muscle for energy if it doesn't have food or drinks for fuel.

You **will** burn slightly more fat if you workout without carbs, but you'll also **lose muscle**. Eat something and you'll still burn plenty of fat but without cannibalizing your hard earned muscle for energy.

Sipping a protein shake before, during, and after your workout sends protein directly to your muscles during your strength training, which brings you faster results.

Finally, the shake will keep your energy levels high, even at the last rep of the last set of your workout. Without fuel, your blood sugar will drop and your energy levels will plummet early in your workout.

Sit Ups Are the Worst Exercise for 6 Pack Abs

You want 6 pack abs so you do endless situps. You want to get rid of your arm fat so you do endless curls. Unfortunately, spot reducing fat in specific areas doesn't work and never has. It's one of the most common fitness myths out there.

Your body pulls fat evenly from every part of your body when you exercise, not specifically from the area worked. So, if you want to get rid of arm fat or love handles, you want exercises that will burn the most calories and fat possible. You burn the most calories by working your largest muscle groups like your chest, back and legs, with exercises like pushups, pullups, squats, lunges and sprints.

Let's say that, even though your overall body fat is low, because of your genes you have love handles or thunder thighs that you want to get rid of. The good news is that, because most of your body fat is located in that one specific area, when you do burn fat, almost all the fat burned will come from that specific area. So to quickly eliminate problem areas, focus on burning the most calories, **not** exercising the specific area in which you want to lose fat.

Lift More, Grow Less!

You want bigger muscles so you work the same muscles every single day to encourage them to grow. You've fallen victim to one of the most common fitness myths. Your muscles do not grow larger in the gym. Your muscles grow larger in bed while you sleep! Muscular contractions from strength training create tiny micro-tears in your muscles. While you sleep and recover, your body repairs the muscles tears and fills the gaps in with new muscle tissue, which makes them stronger. This recovery process takes an average of 24-72 hours. If you keep tearing the same muscles faster than they can recover, the muscles will get weaker over time, not stronger. The more severely you work a muscle, the more time it will take to repair.

Normal daily activities like walking around, light jogs, and housework can be fully recovered from in a single night's sleep, but, you do not want to do intense strength training on the same muscle groups day after day without rest. Doing as many heavy bench presses or heavy dead lifts as you can every day will tear the muscle apart faster than it can heal, and ultimately leave you weaker, not stronger.

If you're still noticeably sore from your last workout, wait to work that muscle again until it feels better. At most, do an "Active Recovery" workout with light weights to pump fresh blood into the muscle. Don't use more than 50% of your normal lifting weight and stop before you hit muscular failure, which is what it's called when you can't do any more repetitions of the exercise with good form.

Your Body Is Your

Castle

Think about your body as a castle you want to build. The exercises you do are your building plans. Your food is the building material. Your sleep is your workers. With any one of the 3 parts missing, you will not be able to build your castle.

Would you ask 2 workers to make you a castle overnight by themselves? That's what you're doing when you follow a really hard workout up with just a few hours of sleep that night.

Would you ask a team of workers to build a tool shed, but then give them enough supplies to build a castle? At the end of the job, there are going to be supplies left over. That's what you're doing when you do a light workout and then eat a huge amount, storing the unused calories as fat.

Would you ask workers to make you a castle out of 10 bricks and a single bag of cement? Despite the workers best intentions, they simply do not have the resources that they need to get the job done. That's what you're doing when you do a heavy workout and get plenty of sleep, but then deprive your body of the nutrients and protein it needs to recover from the workout. No matter how good your workout, or how complete your sleep and recovery, without adequate nutrition, you will not be able to build a better body.

Would you tell your workers to start building the roof of the castle before the initial foundation had been poured? That's what you're doing when you work a muscle before it has fully recovered from the last workout.

Would you hand workers some bricks and mortar and walk away without giving them any clue what you want them to build? The supplies will just sit there for later, since the workers don't know what you want them to do with it. That's what happens when you get plenty of sleep and food, but don't workout and show your body how you want it to get stronger.

What do you think would be the best way to build your castle? You'd need to provide a clear plan to a full team of workers and give them all the resources they need. That's what you do when you work out hard, eat right, and get enough rest. Your builders, plan, and building supplies must all be balanced to build your body into your perfect castle.

Your Body Is Your Masterpiece

If you don't love your body, you don't have to settle for what you have. Your body is your masterpiece, your physical ideal of perfection. It is yours to change however you like. You deserve to look in the mirror and love everything you see.

"Carpenters bend wood, fletchers bend arrows; wise men

fashion themselves." - Buddha

Think of your body like a Greek sculpture. Your strength training instructs the sculptor where to add the clay, while your fat burning exercise carves clay away to reveal the form beneath.

Your food is the clay that will be added to the sculpture's muscles and fuel the fat burning exercise that will remove clay from unwanted spots.

When you go to sleep, the sculptor comes in, adds, and removes the clay as you instructed him, working his magic. Night after night of sleep, your sculptor works on your body. Every day the sculpture is refined and improved by adding more clay to desirable areas, while undesirable areas are sculpted away. Every night, the sculpture improves, and every time you workout, you give the sculptor fresh guidance on where you want clay added and removed to build your masterpiece.

"Good bodybuilders have the same mindset as a sculptor.

You look in the mirror and say, 'I need a little more deltoids, a little more shoulders to get the proportions right.' So, you exercise and put those deltoids on. While an artist would just slap some clay on his statue, we do it the harder way and sculpt our actual bodies." - Arnold Schwarzenegger

Stop Soreness!

I've got some great secrets to make muscle soreness a thing of the past. I recommend doing cardio, such as light jogging or swimming for 10-20 minutes after strength training. Stretch 10-20 minutes after strength training. Drink lots of water and electrolyte (potassium and sodium) enriched sports drinks during or after your workout. Have a carbohydrate and protein shake within 20-45 minutes of strength training. Cut down on the number of sets, reps, or weights.

Any time you are starting a new workout, or throwing much higher demands upon your body than it's used to, you are likely to be sore. By slowly increasing your workouts overtime, you will minimize this.

If you are used to doing 2 sets of 10 pushups in your workouts, next week go for 2 sets of 11 pushups, not 10 sets of 15 pushups, unless you don't mind being seriously sore. Get 8+ hours of sleep after you workout to give your body plenty of time to repair and grow your muscles.

Avoid alcohol, it slows your metabolism down, reduces testosterone, slows protein processing, which slows muscle recovery.

If you want to keep your Fat Bank vault door open, limit your intense workouts to 30-60 minute sessions, or you will be inadvertently slamming your fat loss door shut. An **"Intense"** workout for me might be impossible for one person and easy for someone else, so it's all relative. Experiment with what works best for you and try to stay within the 30-60 minute range.

During workouts, sipping juice, a sports drink like Gatorade, Powerade, or a protein shake helps keep you energized and reassures your body that their are calories coming in and that starvation is not a serious threat. You are telling your body that it can hold off from throwing the brakes on your calorie burning by dunking you in a cortisol bath.

If you do have a particularly long or intense workout and want to knock your cortisol levels back down, the best way is to eat. Your muscles are hungry for energy and protein, and with nothing else to digest for fuel, they will actually cannibalize themselves for energy.

Make Boring Workouts a Thing of the Past!

If you find working out boring, here are few quick easy tips to help: Mix up the exercises. Go with a friend. Get re-motivated with a specific goal (sculpt a body part, set a new personal weight lifting record, improve your speed or strength for a sport, fit into your old jeans, hit a new personal record, get in a contest with a friend to lose the most weight, get a 6 pack for beach season, etc).

Take pictures of yourself with your shirt off to show your progress. Get pictures of goals your working toward, old pictures of yourself, and/or pictures of models or celebrities with the body that you would **like** to have.

Use workout mixes, audio books, or podcasts during workouts. Do compound exercises so that you can work multiple groups at once and finish quickly. Each set after the first gives less returns, so it's okay to do just 1-2 sets (3-4 is slightly better, but not much).

Choose workouts you'll enjoy, such as sports, running outside, swimming, or strength training in the specific areas that will improve your skills in the hobbies you enjoy (for example, squats to improve your jumps on the basketball court). The only workouts that you'll stick with long term are the ones that you enjoy.

Try to workout during the time of day when your energy levels are highest. Just get started, even if don't feel like it.

After 10 minutes of light cardio and breaking a sweat, my adrenaline is flowing and I feel 10x more energetic than I did when I started. Do the same.

Write down workout records so that 1) you can see your progress and 2) you are always motivated to beat your last personal best.

You need to write down solid and realistic short-term and long-term goals that get you excited. Take pictures of yourself and write down goals so that you can check back in a few weeks or months and see your progress.

Don't Deprive Yourself!

Reward Yourself!

To give your body the nutrients it needs to recover from it's workout, and kung fu chop your cortisol, you should eat a protein and carbohydrate rich snack or shake within 20-45 minutes of finishing your workout. If it has some sugar in it, that is fine because your body is so starved for energy that it will immediate take that energy and use it, without storing any of it as fat.

Studies have shown snacks and shakes like this can be just as effective for strength and workout gains before your workout as after, and are used as fuel to help you workout even harder instead of being stored as fat.

This all makes sense, if you think back to your real-life bank account. When are you least likely to save the cash someone gives you? It's probably when they give it to you right before or right after you make a big purchase. You'll use the cash either on the purchase or to pay off the big bill on your credit card that you just racked up!

Time your major deposits for right before or right after a major withdrawal so that it balances out and doesn't end up being stored in the Fat Bank. When you get your pay check for the month on the first of the month and then rent, loans, insurance and utility bills are all due, it feels like you never got your pay check at all, right? It makes it hard to save, but that's exactly what you want, since saved calories become fat and you're trying to **avoid** savings.

If you feel deprived, you will #11 be miserable and #2 be unlikely to stick to it. Tell a kid that he can't play with a particular toy, and it's all he'll want. Likewise, take someone who wants to lose weight and tell them that they **can't** have chocolate or a steak and they'll think about it much more frequently than if it wasn't forbidden.

So, we're going to avoid this completely; nothing is forbidden. You can eat whatever you want and you can eat however much you want, but you just can't do both.

Have a serious craving for sweets? Go for it! Just make sure you just get one portion, put in on a plate, put the container back away and don't go for seconds.

Want to eat tons for entertainment or relaxation? Stick to healthy stuff. I try to think in terms of balance, so, if I want to take in some huge indulgence but I don't want to gain weight, I will exercise to burn the calories off before or after the meal. This way, I break even or end up burning a little more than I take in.

Promising yourself that you can only have the treat if you burn it off tends to either de-motivate you from wanting the treat, or highly motivate you to exercise! Bundling workouts with rewards as a package deal is a great way to guarantee that you finally get that workout in that you keep putting off!

#4 Sleep & You:

How to Open Your Fat Bank Vault

"O bed! O bed! delicious bed! That heaven upon earth to the weary head." - Thomas Hood

"No day is so bad it can't be fixed with a nap." - Carrie Snow

The Power of the Pillow

The vast majority of people do not get enough sleep. Sleep deprivation dunks you in a cortisol jacuzzi that slows your metabolism to a crawl and makes it almost impossible to lose fat because your body is in a hibernation mode which causes it to burn calories as slowly as possible. As long as you are sleep deprived, your Fat Bank vault is slammed close, and you can't make any withdrawals. I will teach you how to open up your Fat Bank vault so you can empty it out!

The Miracle Drug

So, what if I told you that there was a miracle drug that was proven to make you happier, more focused, and more energized? What if it also kept you healthy, strong, and lean? What if it was completely free, everyone could take it, and it had no negative side effects? Would you take it?

I'm happy to say, there actually is such a thing, it's called sleep! Increasing and improving your sleep is the single most powerful step that you can take to keep your Fat Bank open for withdrawals and improve your overall quality of life.

Sleep deprivation tosses you into a dank river of cortisol. Some people need a little more or less sleep, but, on average, children and teenagers need 8-10 hours a night and adults need about 8. If you think you need less, there's an easy way to find out.

For a few days, go to sleep 8 hours before your morning alarm is scheduled to go off. If you consistently wake up more than a few minutes before your alarm goes off, then the number of hours you've slept is all you normally need. If your alarm consistently interrupts your sleep and you are tempted to hit the snooze button or smash your alarm with a sledge hammer, then you need more than 8 hours.

Most people don't get as much sleep as they need and they pay for it. Your body produces testosterone, processes protein, burns fat, and repairs itself while you sleep. If this process is cut short, your body and mind will not function at their best.

Think of it as trying to take your Indy 500 car back on the race track before your pit crew has a chance to put your last wheel on! Your car is back on the race track, but sparks are flying off your axle and you're not getting nearly the acceleration or control you should be getting since you are missing your 4th tire! If you get less sleep than you need, you will have less mental focus, less energy, lower testosterone, and much higher cortisol levels.

Even if you have trouble sleeping, there are a ton of fast, free, easy, and effective solutions that will help you sleep so you can keep your cortisol levels low and your energy levels sky high!

When Did It Get to Be 3 AM?

If you find yourself getting caught up in things like books, movies, web surfing, or anything else and staying up past your bed time, set a hard deadline that at a certain time you will stop whatever you're doing and go to bed. Personally, even if I have the genuine intention of doing this, I'll still find myself playing a video game at 9 PM, then look up at the clock to notice that it somehow became 4 AM, and I have to work in the morning!

I know I'm not alone, and I've found one simple technique that has completely eliminated this problem for me. Most of us set alarms to let us know when we need to get up in the morning. Go ahead and do the same thing at night, set a sleep alarm for when you want to quit whatever you are doing and go to bed. If you need to take a minute, save your game, finish the page of your book, or say good night to your friends, that's fine, but quit what you're doing and get ready for bed ASAP.

I call this my pumpkin alarm. Cinderella's magic carriage turns into a pumpkin at midnight. Likewise, when my alarm goes off, no matter where I am or what I'm doing, I magically turn into a pumpkin and have to go to bed.

Stay Regular

However much sleep we get, or don't get, the sleep will go a lot further if we go to sleep and wake up around the same time everyday. If you get 8 hours one day sleeping from 12 AM-8 AM, and 8 hours the next day sleeping from 4 AM-12 PM, you are going to feel off. The closer you can get to a consistent waking and sleeping schedule, the better rested and more refreshed you will feel.

Cozy Conditioning

If you only use your bed for sleeping and sex, you will condition your body to automatically relax when you crawl in. If you watch movies, read books and do homework in bed, you will condition yourself to stay awake there, and it will be much harder to sleep in it at night.

The Zen of Relaxation

You will have an easier time sleeping if you don't consume any caffeine, sugar, or heavy meals within 3-6 hours of sleep; they will stimulate your system and keep you wired. When you do get into bed, don't start any stimulating activities like video games or action movies; you want to slow your system down to get it ready for rest. Do light stretching, take a hot shower, put on soothing music, read something boring, pray or meditate, and try to clear your mind.

If you have a lot of things on your mind that you need to take care of tomorrow, or that you can't stop thinking about, write them down to clear your head and you can take care of them in the morning.

Wear Yourself Out

You can be mentally exhausted but still completely fresh physically. If you've barely moved around that day and it's hard to convince your body that it's done anything it needs to rest from. Exercising and strength training during the day will help you sleep better at night since your body will be ready to recover from the work it's done.

Getting this deep sleep will give you better focus, more energy, and lower cortisol levels during the day

and will help in one other very important way.
When people are sleepy and sluggish they crave
sugar, caffeine, and other stimulants to wake up and
energize their systems. If your system already had
enough sleep, it's much easier to skip these
indulgences since your already feeling mentally
alert.

When you're tired, your body also produces much
higher levels of a chemical called ghrelin, which is
what makes you feel hungry. For all the reasons I've
explained, getting more sleep is the single most
important thing you can do to change your body.

#5 Stress &

You: *How to Keep Your Fat Bank Vault Open for Withdrawals*

"A crust eaten in peace is better than a banquet partaken in anxiety." - Aesop

"Food for the body is not enough. There must be food for the soul." - Dorothy Day

Stress Makes You Fat

Physical stress isn't the only thing that kicks your cortisol production into high gear. Mental and emotional stress do too. Your systems senses that you're feeling uneasy and threatened in some way. It thinks your food supply may be threatened.

Maybe you're actually stressed because someone mugged you and stole your watch, you were passed over for a promotion at work, or gas is $4 at the pump and rising. Whatever it is, your body doesn't know any of that. It just knows that your producing the same stress chemicals in your brain that your ancestors produced when someone bigger threatened them, when their food stash was stolen, when they weren't able to catch anything on their hunt and came home empty handed, or worse, when they felt hopelessly lost, wandering through a barren wasteland where edible plants were few and far between.

Your body doesn't know the difference between emotional, intellectual, and physical stress. It interprets all of them as threats to its food supply and kicks cortisol production into high gear to slam your Fat Bank vault door closed.

As a result, you use calories as slowly as possible and can survive long enough to make it to your next meal. Spending your life stressed out means spending your life soaking in a cortisol bath, which slows your fat burning to a crawl.

The reason people try to lose fat is because they believe they will be happier if they do. Since happiness is the end goal anyway, and stress is the enemy of happiness, let me present a few strategies to increase your happiness and manage your stress. Fortunately some of the very best ways to minimize stress are eating healthy, sleeping well and exercising, which we have already covered in the previous areas.

As Albert Einstein said, "Life is like riding a bicycle.

To keep your balance you must keep moving."
Besides exercise, nutrition, and sleep, there are many
other lifestyle-focused techniques that will lower
your stress, lower your cortisol, keep your Fat Bank
vault open for withdrawals, and, most importantly,
make you happier!

Don't Be a Square Peg Shoved into a Round Hole

What makes you feel your very best? What
experiences or activities leave you feeling most
energized, motivated, and positive? Conversely,
what makes you feel your very worst? What
experiences or activities leave you feeling the most
beat down, discouraged and drained?

These specific uppers and downers are unique to

every individual. The things that make one person feel their best, will make another feel their worst, like country or heavy metal music! You might love painting, but hate number crunching, or love writing murder mysteries but hate doing housework. Most people have many different uppers and downers, make sure you think of at least three of each.

Now, ask yourself if there's any way that you can squeeze more upper into your day and can beg or bargain your way out of some of your downers. Are there people whose skills would better suit your downers, or who would actually enjoy it? Can you trade the downers to other people for things you are happy to do in return? Maybe you love baking, and your neighbor loves doing the lawn care you can't stand. Could you trade weekly batches of sweet treats in exchange for your neighbor mowing your lawn?

Do the downers even have to get done, would anybody mind if they were skipped? Maybe you scrub and dust your house weekly and no one else would even notice if you cleaned every few months instead.

Can you hire out the work affordably or buy products that will do your work for you? Maybe your daughter would be just as happy to get a $10 halloween outfit from Wal-Mart, instead of the hand stitched costume you've been slaving away on for weeks?

Are their any tools or strategies you can use to make the downer more pleasant? Personally, I don't like driving in areas that I'm not familiar with because I get lost easily. Fortunately, I live in an era of high-quality GPS systems that cost under $100, which saves me endless stress and anxiety on the road. Instead of cursing myself for not having a better sense of direction, I can enjoy the drive, confident that I will reach my destination. My GPS transforms my downer into an upper. Is there a product or trade you can make like this, to avoid or improve a downer in your own life?

Prime Time

We are all human. No matter how hard we push ourselves, we each have finite focus and limited mental energy. By admitting this, we free ourselves to strategically match our highest energy levels to our greatest challenges.

I call the time when I'm feeling my best, my **prime time**. For some people they are at their freshest after a workout, or first thing in the morning after coffee. Other people are at their best after work or even right before bed. Whenever your feel at your mental and emotional best, don't waste that time on mindless tasks. Take on the great challenges that would be almost impossible when you're tired.

At best, each of us only gets an hour or two of prime time a day. Don't waste it on busy work you could do when you're tired. Write that carefully written e-mail. Make the difficult but necessary phone call. Work on your book manuscript. Do your taxes. Laundry, vacuuming, and grocery shopping are busy work for some people, but if you are new to those tasks or detest them, it's fair game to reserve them for **prime time** when you can fully psych yourself up to the challenge.

Do not watch TV, goof off, play video games, drink, surf the net or read comic books. Invest your prime time in difficult pursuits that require your peak mental focus.

Doing your Calculus homework might be unthinkable at 11 PM after a long hard day. Try it while sipping your morning coffee at 10 AM after a good night's sleep, breakfast, and a great workout. If you feel like I do about Calculus, you still won't enjoy it, but the exact same work will suddenly be **much** more bearable.

Throughout your day whenever you are feeling at your best, tackle your hardest mental and emotional challenges. Reserve busy work that you can do on autopilot for when you are tired and not feeling your freshest. You already have all the focus you need to wildly succeed. You owe it to yourself to use your **prime time** on worthy challenges instead of letting it go to waste on tasks you can do anytime.

What's the Magic Word?

There is no one secret to happiness, but I can confidently tell you the one guaranteed secret to misery. Trying to please everybody all the time. Everyone wants different, incompatible, unreasonable, and often contradictory things. No matter what you do someone will be left disappointed. "Hey Samantha, while I appreciate you canceling your anniversary date with your husband last night, so you could stay up all night building this fully functional jet pack prototype, I really don't care for your choice of color, can you do it over in paisley?" Some people are going to be left unsatisfied no matter what you do. Given that, there's no sense getting stressed out when it won't make any difference either way.

There are some things that you must do, and some things that you enjoy doing. To make the most time possible for those 2 things (I guarantee there are more of both than any of us will ever have time for), say no. Politely apologize and explain that you'd like to help but your time is limited and you've already committed to taking care of other things first.

Be firm, stand your ground, and you will be surprised how easy it becomes to say no. Plus, you will suddenly have much more time to work on the projects that will have the greatest impact on your life!

If You Find Yourself at the Bottom of a Hole, Stop Digging

"The definition of insanity is doing the same thing over and over again and expecting different results." - Albert Einstein

There is a psychological term called rumination, it rhymes with ruination and leads directly to it. It means going over the same stressful thoughts over and over again in your head. Now there's nothing wrong with thinking about something, but repeating the same thought process 1000 times doesn't accomplish any more than going over it once.

It's the mental equivalent of walking in circles, and all it does is waste your precious mental and emotional energy that you could be spending on better things. Time spent worrying is time wasted. If it is something you really want to work out and change, sit down, write out the situation, and either make your decision, or figure out what information you still require to make a correct fully informed decision in the future.

If you keep digging yourself into a stress hole by repeating the same thoughts, please stop. You can't dig yourself out of a hole. When you have a song stuck in your head, if you try not to think about it, it will keep popping back into your head. Your best bet is to listen to a new song to refocus your mind on something new. Likewise, when you catch yourself ruminating, don't try to think your way out of the problem. Try to absorb yourself in a different topic completely and change your tune!

Want to Want What You Want

"Knowing yourself is the beginning of all wisdom." - Aristotle

The happiest people want to want what they want. I've known plenty of people who maintained 6 pack abs but were miserable, because what they really wanted was to eat pizza and ice cream. I've known nationally ranked athletes that were miserable, they were sick of non-stop training and competing. What they really wanted was to pursue hobbies and a life beyond sports. Likewise, we all know people who eat whatever they want, but are miserable because what they really want deep down is to have a healthy body they are proud of. So, what do you really want?

If you really want 6 pack abs, to run a marathon, or

increase your bench press, you need to work, fight and sweat for those goals. Every sacrifice will bring you closer to victory and make you happier. If you really want to relax on the couch and indulge in every food under the sun, please enjoy yourself guilt free and live it up!

People get in trouble focusing on what they want to want. They wish they wanted to work out but they don't. They wish they were motivated to lose fat, but they aren't. They are happy the way they are and don't think it's worth changing their lifestyle. To me, that's okay. As long as you're doing what makes you happy, you're doing something right!

Don't worry about what you want to want. Focus on exploring and accepting what it is that you really want. Don't fight it or kick yourself for it. Embrace your desires and take pride in wanting to want what you want. Your goals may change over time. What you really want may be a balanced life including fitness and indulgence. There's no one right goal for everyone. Figure out what it is that you really want, live it, love it, own it and proudly want to want what you want.

"Happiness is when what you think, what you say, and what you do are in harmony." – Mahatma Gandhi

One Thing at a Time

One of the keys to getting a lot done is to do very little. We are not wired to multi-task. Every distraction and separate task we throw at our minds slows us down. Imagine a small compact car driving down the road. But it doesn't just have to haul it's own weight with it's tiny engine. It has to tow another compact car behind it. It will struggle to accelerate, brake dangerously slowly and go at a snail's pace when attempting to climb any hill.

Your brain is not a tow truck, or a mack truck, it is a car to get you from one problem to one solution.

Do one thing and give it your complete focus. You will be blown away by how much more quickly you get things done.

It's easy for people to feel pressured to do 10 things at once because they have a lot to do. But, the difference between the people who manage their time well and those who don't is whether or not they accept the fact that every single one of us has more to do than we could ever hope to complete. That doesn't make us slow, stupid, or lazy; it's simply a fact of modern life.

Unfortunately, because we have too many things to do, it's easy to feel overwhelmed, or try to make everything our top priority. However, the problem with that is that it also means that you've simultaneously made everything your lowest priority. But, just because we can't do **everything** doesn't mean that we can't do **anything**!

Ask yourself what specific change would have the

biggest impact on both your professional and personal life, and spend more focused time working on that. You will have dozens of interruptions and emergencies begging to break your focus during the day. But urgent issues are not always high impact issues. Just because something or someone asks for your immediate attention doesn't mean the task is particularly important, or that it will take you closer to your goal. If these urgent issues will not have a greater impact on your life then the important project you are working towards, then put them off, find someone else who can deal with them, or just let them go.

There are only so many hours in the day, and you've made peace with that, putting your time and focus where it can do the absolute most good. No one could ever ask you for more.

To often, we spend our time on the same problems that keep springing up over and over again. Picture yourself in a flooded basement, up to your waist in water and frantically trying to bail the place out with a bucket. Most of us spend most of our time feeling this way, buried under our immediate work emergencies and family obligations.

Water keeps pouring down just as fast as you can bail it out, and you feel like you aren't making any real progress. Suddenly, you realize that until you fix the **cause** of the water you will be stuck trying to fix the **symptoms** of the water forever. You throw your bucket down and run upstairs. You find the leaky pipe on the 1st floor that is causing the basement flood, turn off the water to the pipe and replace it with a new part.

Instead of being locked in an eternal struggle with the symptoms of the problem, you have conquered the root cause itself and can move on with your life. When you empty out the basement you can be confident that this will be the last time you ever have to deal with the problem, and that it won't be coming back.

You Deserve the Best

Some people make the room feel emptier when they enter it. They feel so insecure and unhappy themselves that they try to put down everyone around them to make themselves feel better. Some people will take your self improvements efforts as a threat that you are too good for them, or as a reminder of how lazy they are.

If your friends and family are perfectly happy with their less than healthy lifestyles, don't try to convert them. It's their lives to lead as they see fit. But, if they are interested in what you're doing, try sharing some of the secrets you've learned in this book with them. Cook for them, exercise with them, and see if they can start enjoying healthier habits with you. If, despite your best efforts, someone keeps disrespecting you or your healthy choices, spend your time with others who respect you and your lifestyle.

Spend your time with people who support you and the positive changes you are trying to make in your life. Look for people who "Think up, not down." If you must spend time with negative people at home or at work, minimize your interactions with them and try to use their negativity to motivate you to prove them wrong. As Walter Gagebot said, "A great pleasure in life is doing what people say you cannot do."

P.E.R.K.

At work and at home, you are spending time on activities that improve your quality of life. You're also doing a lot of things that simply must be done. But, if you're like most people, you're also spending much of your time on things that aren't doing much for you. You don't need to squeeze more **into** your day, your goal is to get more **out** of your day.

You don't want to **spend** time, you want to **invest** it in the activities that will give you the best return and make you feel your best. Write up a quick list of your daily activities and P.E.R.K. it! Go through and choose the activities you can Postpone, Eliminate, Reduce or Keep. You will be amazed at how this one change will free up your time and focus your time and energy on the activities that will improve your life the most.

Make Everyday Your Masterpiece

Before you go to sleep, or when you wake up in the morning, take a few minutes to think about what you'd like to happen that day. If you could accomplish anything that day, what would you do? What would you feel proud of as you lay down to sleep that night? As you mentally envision your masterpiece, there are just a few requirements.

Under Your Control

You have to choose activities that are under your direct control. You could make a doctor's appointment, ask that cute life guard out on a date, get your hair cut, shop for groceries, ask your boss for a promotion, paint for an hour, or cook a healthy gourmet meal.

Do not assemble your masterpiece with activities that are either unrealistic or out of your control. Do not plan on building a spaceship or achieving world peace. There's nothing wrong with being optimistic, but don't include any action that you wouldn't feel comfortable betting $10 that you could do. If you haven't gone running for years, plan on a 1 mile jog, not a 26 mile marathon. If you're a musician, try to come up with a new song tomorrow, not a whole new CD.

Sharpen Your Saw

Your masterpiece must include some "you time".
Slip in something you will look forward to,
something that makes you smile. No matter what,
you must include at least 30 minutes doing a specific
activity that makes you feel good. It can be
catching up with an old friend on the phone, playing
video games, reading, jogging, playing piano,
watching a tv show, meditating, doing yoga, or
anything you want that is both enjoyable and purely
for you!

This might sound simple, but you wouldn't believe
how many people never make any time for
themselves. Recharging your battery this way is
absolutely essential to be at your best the other 23
1/2 hours of the day!

If you want to contribute to your family and co-workers, do them a favor, and take some time to have some fun. In Stephen Covey's best selling book *The Seven Habits of Highly Effective People,* he refers to this essential technique as sharpening your saw.

If you are cutting down a tree, over time your saw will dull, and you will just be pointlessly rubbing the smooth metal against the bark. After countless sweat-drenched hours, you realize no matter how hard you work, or how many hours you put in, you will not be able to make any progress cutting through the tree. So, you stop cutting the tree, sit down on on a moss-covered rock, and spend your next 30 minutes sharpening your saw until it's razor sharp.

You take your newly sharpened saw and again begin cutting the tree. Unlike before, where your best efforts seemed to accomplish nothing, now you are seeing fast results. Within a few minutes, you've cut completely through the tree and your task is completed. You realize that you would never have been able to do it as quickly or as easily if you hadn't taken some time away from work to sharpen your saw.

"Time you enjoy wasting, was not wasted." – John Lennon

You need to sharpen your saw for your physical, emotional, and mental needs to be met, to do your best work and treat your friends, classmates, co-workers and family right. This time is not selfish. The better you take care of yourself and the better you feel, the better you will treat everyone else, and the more energy you'll have to give to them.

The thing to feel guilty about is **not** taking the time to take care of yourself. If you're not taking "you time", you're not giving your friends and family your best. Many people feel like they somehow "shouldn't need it." But the truth is, most people need it just to function at all, and absolutely everyone needs it to be at their best.

Never Stop Growing

"Do today what others will not, so that you may do tomorrow what others cannot." - Anonymous

None of us want to look back 10 years from now and realize we have nothing to show for the past decade. We haven't learned new skills, haven't improved our circumstances and haven't made new friends. Yet, many of us find ourselves in that exact situation. If we aren't careful with how we spend our time, it will flow through our fingers as if we were juggling sand.

"Do not squander time time for that is the stuff life is made of." - Benjamin Franklin

Your masterpiece for every day should include at least 30 minutes of doing something difficult that will help you grow. You could study statistics, talk to your kids about the birds and bees, clean the basement, expand your Spanish vocabulary, work on your taxes, or do any of the countless things that you would love to put off, but would also love to have finished and off your to do list! 30 minutes of anything won't kill us, and, as you put time into these areas, they will quickly improve and stop stressing you out!

These 30 minutes a day gives us a chance to chisel away at those tough tasks we've been putting off, and break them off into manageable bite-size chunks so that overtime they get done. Just 1/2 an hour a day is 10,950 minutes a year. Imagine how much you could achieve, and how far you could move yourself forward if you invest that time in yourself?

#6 Habits &

You: *How to Automate Your Fat Bank Withdrawals*

"First we make our habits, then our habits make us." - Charles C. Noble

"Motivation is what gets you started. Habit is what keeps you going." - Jim Rohn

Discipline Is a Muscle

"I can accept failure, everyone fails at something. But I can't accept not trying." - Michael Jordan

Even if you fully understand these strategies, you may assume that you still don't have the inner reserves of strength necessary to change your lifestyle and switch to healthy routines. You absolutely without question **do** have what it takes.

If you told me ten years ago that I would be giving fitness advice, I would have laughed in your face! I was a pack a day smoker, weighed over 250 pounds, was the last pick for any gym class and couldn't do a pushup. Healthy moderation meant getting the large movie theater popcorn with extra butter and a large soda, instead of springing for the XXL size.

So what inspired me to change? I found a physical activity I actually liked. I started learning about break dancing and taking classes. I was so focused on practicing the moves that I didn't even notice all the weight that was disappearing.

I ended up starting a street dance online store selling training videos, competitions and protective gear. We're the largest of our kind with over 1000+ videos. The site is CypherStyles.com if you want to check it out or look for how to street dance videos, gear or hip hop aerobic workouts.

Street dance was what did it for me, but the prospect of spinning on your head may not particularly excite you. That's okay, everyone has or can find some physical activity they enjoy.

Most people assume to get fit they need to lift weights or hit the treadmills and elliptical, but your body doesn't care how you move, just **that** you move. The best exercise plan is the one you'll actually do, which for many people is the one that doesn't feel like exercise. If I go to dance, I look forward to it and have a great time. It's not a chore to go, and I'm self-motivated because I enjoy it.

If you try a class you hate that burns plenty of calories, you'll get fed up with it and quit after a week (or if you're like me you'll quit mid-way through the class). If you don't like it, you won't do it.

Keep taking new classes and activities until you find one that you enjoy. It doesn't matter if it is the most intense or burns the most calories. If it's something you enjoy, you'll stick with it, enjoy yourself, and see dramatic results over time. As Aristotle famously said, "We are what we repeatedly do. Excellence, then, is not an act, but a habit."

Try Different

"The usual mantra is to 'try harder'. Trying harder is impossible when you're already trying as hard as you can. But you can always try different." - Seth Godin

I tried many, many times to change my diet and exercise habits unsuccessfully, but every attempt brought be a little closer to my goals. Every time I went a little longer before breaking my diet, I gained a little more discipline and self respect. Mistakes are how we learn what works and what doesn't. It's proven that for both smokers and over-eaters the more times they attempt to quit, the more likely they are to quit for good.

"An expert is a man who has made all the mistakes which can be made, in a narrow field." - Niels Bohr

If skipping desert today is an unthinkable feat, that's okay, just try to leave a forkful left on your plate instead of finishing it. Focus on making slow baby steps over time.

Some people think they don't have any discipline or self control, but there's an easy way to prove that isn't true. Normally, left to it's own devices, your body will breathe continuously, but, if you focus, you can stop your lungs and hold your breath. Even the most undisciplined among us can hold our breath and exert control over ourselves to some extent. It's all about taking control and pushing our limits, wherever they happen to be.

Discipline is a mental muscle and, just like your physical muscles, it gets stronger over time as you work it. "I might only be able to jog a few blocks before I get winded today, but next week I'll be able to run a mile, and in a few months I'll run a 5K!" "I might not have enough discipline to skip desert completely, but I'll split it with a friend today and have some fresh fruit for desert tomorrow."

As you make these healthy choices, even if they require a Herculean amount of effort at first, they become easier and easier until they are completely automatic and require no effort at all. At first our best might not be good enough, but as we stick with our new lifestyle, our best gets better and we can handle anything.

"What we hope ever to do with ease, we must learn first to do with diligence." - Samuel Johnson

We Do What We Like, We Like What We Do

We build our routines to include the activities we enjoy and our routines comfort us like familiar friends.   In short, we do what we like and we like what we do!

"Man cannot discover new oceans until he has the courage to lose the sight of the shore." - André Gide

Changing your routine is like taking a massive locomotive speeding down a track and forcing it to grind to a halt and slowly reverse direction. This act is difficult and requires a great deal of conscious effort, particularly as you slow the train and then built momentum the other way.

But, in the words of Winston Churchill, "When you're going through hell, keep going." In fact, once you have built up the momentum, it becomes just as easy to maintain as your current routines. It gets easier and easier after that first initial push, until your newly generated momentum takes hold of you completely. The momentum that makes it hard to change your unhealthy routines is the exact same momentum that will make it easy to maintain these healthy habits once you begin them.

Progress, Not Perfection

"Ever tried. Ever failed. No matter. Try again. Fail again. Fail better." - Samuel Beckett"

You will make more progress in your goals in 3 months of minor healthy lifestyle adjustments than you will in 3 weeks of incredibly intense training.

Most people try to transform their bodies overnight, hate the brutal training and dieting, and give up because it's so unpleasant. You're much better off making small improvements that you can stick with; that's all it takes to see permanent changes in your body.

Reaching your goals just requires that you focus on "Progress, Not Perfection." No one takes care of his or her body perfectly, just try to make the changes that will be the easiest for you.

Maybe you have a sweet tooth, but you love team sports. Great, keep enjoying treats, but go join a recreational sports team. Maybe you love strength training but hate cardio. No problem, focus on strength training. Increase your muscle mass so you can permanently increase your metabolism and burn more fat. Maybe you hate working out but you are happy eating healthy. Great, cut down on the fat and sugar in your diet and start going for walks and doing more active work around the house.

All these changes will help you drain your Fat Bank in ways that are easy and even fun! The right plan is the one you will actually do, so focus on the food, exercise, sleep, and stress management changes that will be the easiest to make. You don't have to do everything, just improve on what you're doing today, stick with it, and you will see huge progress.

Your Effort Today Is Your Body Tomorrow

The biggest difference between people who succeed and people who fail is not a difference in potential, or even a difference in discipline. People who succeed realize that doing anything new is tough. They accept that doing something new will be difficult, but, will gradually get easier over time.

The activity is not hard because the person is weak, uncoordinated, stupid, or bad. It is hard because doing anything new is difficult and takes time. Most people who fail do not understand this. When something is hard for them, they take that as a sign that it just wasn't meant for them. They assume that the skill must come easy for anyone meant to do it. Since it's hard, they assume that it will always be hard. They don't realize that it's hard because it's new and that in time it will become easy.

Most people just assume if they are bad at something they will always be bad at it or that they just aren't cut out for it. When you see someone do a backflip effortlessly, or draw a beautiful picture, it's easy to assume that those skills are the result of inherent natural talent. They can do those things effortlessly, so, if you have to strain to attempt them, you must be doing something wrong, right?

The truth is this: "Being great is easy. Becoming great is hard." Over time, challenges that are currently impossible for us will become easy, but that path requires time and effort for **everyone** including the best of the best. Michael Jordan's basketball ability didn't just happen, he had to work tirelessly to achieve it. Bill Gates wasn't born talented with computers, he spent every free moment of his childhood and teenage years working on his computer programming skills.

Who you are today doesn't have to limit or define your tomorrow. Everything gets better with practice. Foster a growth mindset and **anything** is possible in your life.

You may or may not be willing to put the time and effort in, and that's completely okay. There are only so many hours in the day and only so many things we can squeeze into our schedules, but nothing is out of your reach if you want it. What was impossible yesterday will be hard today and effortless tomorrow. All that effort will pay off. Remember, your effort today is your body tomorrow.

Get Specific

It's great to have a goal or a dream, that's where it all starts. But gazing at the moon, and wondering what it would look like up close is very different from building a rocket ship, and flying up to actually walk on its surface. It's the difference between dreaming of California sunsets, and booking your plane ticket and photo session on the Golden Gate Bridge.

When you have a general goal, try to get as specific as you can and break it into steps. If you don't know exactly where you want to go, you will waste a lot of time going in the wrong direction. If your goal is abstract, it's hard to know how to get there, or if you're off track.

Make your goals as specific and quantifiable as possible, write them down, include a deadline, and at least a few of the steps that will bring you closer to that goal. If it didn't work out, check back and see what needs to be changed so that it works next time.

Maybe you had trouble reaching your goal to work up to 20 straight pushup because it didn't really inspire you. You either need to find a goal that excites you or you need to free up more time to work towards a motivating goal you already have. To decide, you need to focus in and choose exactly what your specific goal is.

Goal Systems

Most people say "I want to get fit" or "I want to lose weight," and they leave it at that. Unfortunately, there is more to achieving a goal than simply stating it. With only a goal and no way to reach it, the goal is never achieved. So, don't just make a goal; make a goal system. Goal systems take you beyond a goal to a structured environment and support system that will continuously guide you to achieve that goal. If you throw a bowling ball down a lane, it might fall into the gutter without ever hitting any pins. If you place bumpers in the gutters, you can't fail. No matter what, your throw will stay out of the gutter and you can't help but knock your pins down and get points. Goal systems do the same thing: they keep you out of trouble, block potential opportunities for failure, and help guide you to victory.

The same habits that will help you achieve your fat loss goals will help you achieve goals in every other aspect of your life. Having a goal is not enough. A goal by itself is just a dream, and we want to make our goals realities. To turn our dreams into reality, we need complete goal systems, and the goal itself is only the beginning. The goal system is the bridge that takes us from where we are to where we want to be.

"All men dream but not equally. Those who dream by night in the dusty recesses of their minds wake in the day to find that it was vanity; but the dreamers of the day are

dangerous, for they may act their dream with open eyes to make it possible." - T.E. Lawrence

A) Goal Selection - Even if you are focused on far-off, long-term goals, break them down into easily achievable short-term goals with specific deadlines. If you don't have a date you want to achieve them by, it's too easy to just keep putting them off.

Losing 50 pounds of fat is good, but it's more realistic to focus on losing two pounds this week. Maybe you want to be able to run a 26 mile marathon. Great! Start with a 3 mile jog today and a 5 mile jog by the end of the month.

Try using one-to-twelve week time ranges for short-term goals. It's hard to motivate yourself for a goal that's further into the future than that. Also, it's best if goals have a true/false element so that you can really chart progress and know that you've achieved it.

"Getting fit" is pretty vague, and it can be hard to know if you've achieved such an unspecific goal. However, dropping your body fat by 2% by the end of the month is both specific and achievable. So to start, each goal should have (1) a short-term goal that can be achieved within 3 months or less, (2) a true/false element and (3) a deadline.

"The odds of hitting a target go up dramatically when you aim at it." - Steve Smith

B) Plan - Let's say that you've completed the first part of goal selection by setting your goal. You want to run a 13.6 mile half marathon by the end of your summer vacation, which gives you three months to train.

"If you're not practicing, somebody else is, somewhere, and he'll be ready to take your job." - Brooks Robinson

Time & Place - What steps do you need to take to achieve your goal? It's proven that setting a time and place beforehand makes it at least 100% more likely that the action will actually be completed. You know you need to put in practice time to achieve your goal, but let's take it further.

You're going to run in the park by your house for 30 minutes every weekday when you come home from your summer job. In addition, one meal each day will be a healthy salad until the end of your summer vacation.

"The difference between a goal and a dream is a deadline." - Steve Smith

Resources - What resources do you need to achieve your goal? If you don't know where to start, find free training guides online. If the pain from your ragged old shoes stops you from training, get a nice new pair of running shoes that will keep you feeling fresh through long training sessions.

Help - Are there people who can help you with

your goal? Maybe you can ask a friend who runs for advice, find a coach, or find a running supply shop in your area?

Progress - What gets measured gets done, so make sure you check back regularly—every week or at least every month—and record your progress. This will keep you motivated, and it will help you see if there is a problem with your plan. Sometimes, even plans with the best intentions just don't work out.

If something isn't working, you want to figure out why and change it. Record the time, distance and frequency of your runs each week. If you miss a run, record that too so that you can catch problems that are getting between you and your goal.
You don't have to write down everything, but you want to have some way of analyzing your progress over time. This way, you can adjust course if you hit a sticking point in your training.

C) Support Structure - None of us have as much

energy or as many hours in the day as we would like. People who achieve their goals are no different; they just accept this and set up a support structure to keep them working toward their goals, even when they would otherwise get distracted and lose focus.

Supplies - Pack up the supplies you need to train (water, music, shoes, and change of clothes) the day before so that you'll have them ready to go.

Competition - Enter a formal half marathon so that you have a reason to train. Or, challenge a friend to run that distance with you on a specific date so that you're both pushing yourselves to win.

Spread The Word - Tell your friends and family about your goals so that you'll have peer pressure keeping you motivated. Run it as a fundraiser and ask friends to sponsor you. You'll want to complete the challenge so that you can raise money for a cause you believe in.

Schedule - Join a running group, a cross country team, or agree to train with a friend for a month so that you're committed to showing up.

Free Up Time - If another hobby, obligation, or habit is getting in the way of your goal, minimize it or cut it out completely. We only have a limited amount of time and energy in the day, and the only way to achieve one thing is to not spend that time working on something else.

D) Action - You've built a full goal system and you have everything you need to make your dream a reality. At this point, you may look at what it will take to reach your goal and decide it's not worth it. Goals aren't reached in isolation; you have to make trade-offs and sacrifices to achieve them. After examining those trade-offs, you may decide the benefits of the goal just aren't worth the trouble. You may need a smaller goal that will be less of a hassle to reach, or a larger goal that is more inspiring. That's okay because it's always better to analyze the pros and cons first. This way, you can make an informed decision, rather then waste weeks or months pursuing the wrong goal.

The goals we choose not to pursue are just as important to our happiness and success as the goals we do pursue. Saying no to the wrong goals, frees us up so that we are available when we find the right goals. If you have found a goal system with both a goal and plan that motivates you, remember that the best plan is only as good as the action that follows it. It's not what you plan to do, but what you actually do that counts. So, follow your goal system and bring your dream to life!

"Some people want it to happen, some wish it would happen, others make it happen." - Michael Jordan

Bad Character or Just

Bad Judgment?

"To err is human, to forgive, divine." Many people feel like they are "bad" when they overeat and feel guilty about their actions. Feeling like they've **done** something bad makes people feel like they **are** bad, which makes them feel weak, powerless, and unable to change or do better. To again quote Henry Ford, "Whether you think you can or you think you can't, you're right."

So, the first step toward breaking that cycle of overeating because you feel bad and feeling bad because you overeat is realizing that there is nothing morally bad about unhealthy eating. Food, exercise, and fat loss are not morally good or evil.

Evil is hurting other people. If you binged on sweets, while on a diet, you haven't hurt anyone. Evil is making the world a worse place. You haven't made the world a worse place with your actions. You haven't caused anyone pain or even done anything irreversible to yourself. What you may have done is made a less than perfect decision, which we all do from time to time, and that is wholly forgivable.

Virtually everyone's goal in life is to do the things that will make him or her the happiest. We do our best to hit a balance of the activities that will make us happy now and happy later. You might enjoy having unprotected sex with strangers today, but you won't enjoy having sexually transmitted diseases tomorrow.

Likewise, you would probably like to be a multi-millionaire when you retire, but it's probably not worth it to you if it means you spend 100 hours a week working and have no social life or family life for the next 50 years. Our goal is to do what will bring us the most happiness in both the long and the short term.

So, if you eat a piece of ice cream cake, you'll feel great while you eat it. It's a scientific fact. The sugar and fat release "comfort chemicals"in your brain, such as serotonin and endorphins, that make you feel happy and relaxed, encouraging you to keep eating the high calorie foods to fill your Fat Bank.

The problem is that, while you feel great for the few minutes that you're eating the food, soon after you regret your indulgence when you crash from the fat and sugar. You regret it, when you look in the mirror and don't like what you see. This regret is a constant and long-term problem that makes you feel bad, while the occasional indulgences that make you feel good only last a few minutes and quickly end in guilt.

So, this process is not evil, but you're trading feeling guilty and bad about your appearance every hour of every day for feeling good from the food you eat for, at the most, a few minutes a day. That's a pretty bad trade. Why do we do it? Because our familiar habits are comforting and easy. Depriving ourselves of what we want and changing our routines is incredibly hard! Fortunately, equipped with the right information and the right attitude, we can build healthier new routines that will make us feel great, and feel great about ourselves!

Food Problem or Food Solution?

Drug relapse rates are extremely high for patients in mandatory drug and alcohol rehabilitation centers. Addictive chemicals are very tough to quit, but long-term failure rates for **optional** drug and alcohol rehabilitation programs are **much** higher than **mandatory** programs.

Both groups have to deal with the same difficult challenge of kicking drugs and alcohol, so why do patients who volunteer for treatment have so much better results?

The reason for the difference is simple: "Change isn't for people that need it, it's for people who want it." As long as people are willing to put up with the consequences of their habits, whether it be poverty, disease, job loss, or family problems, they will not change.

Why would they? They'd rather put up the with the drawbacks of the situation that they are in, than switch to one they perceive as even worse, such as life without that chemical. It's a sad situation, but it is a logical choice. They will not be able to make a permanent change until they decide that the drawbacks of the chemical outweigh the benefits, and they'd be better off without it. It may still take some time and some failed attempts before they quit for good, but this change in perspective must take place to leave the habit behind.

The same principles apply to food. Most people that have issues with overeating claim that they have a "Food Problem" when what they really have is a

"Food Solution." When you're lonely, bored, sad, stressed, or tired, eating makes you feel better. It's a reliable foundation that you can count on to support you during difficult times. Food is a solution for them, so you can't take that away without a new solution to take it's place.

You can't kick the legs out from under a table and expect it to stand, you must replace overeating with different supportive activities, or else, like the legless table, you will collapse. You will either be deeply stressed or go back to indulging in your unhealthy habits. The only way to prevent this is to find new supports that are consistent with your new healthy lifestyle.

"A nail is driven out by another nail. Habit is overcome by habit." - Desiderius Erasmus

Fortunately, if you're read the rest of Empty Your Fat Bank then the the most powerful ways to consistently improve your mood and quality of life will be very familiar to you. Eat healthy, exercise, sleep well, and take time to de-stress. These are not only the best way to improve your quality of life and consistently feel good, they are also the best way to easily say no to unhealthy temptations because you'll be feeling so good that you won't need them!

Make an I.M.P.A.C.T.

The IMPACT process is a great habit to achieve any goal, be it physical, professional, or personal. Robert Pagliarini, author of *The Other 8 Hours*, recommends structuring the things you want to accomplish as IMPACT goals. What is the difference between a plain old ordinary goal and an IMPACT goal?

Inspiring - The biggest reason people fail to reach their goals is not because there is anything wrong with them but because there goal wasn't right for them. If I decide tomorrow that I'm going to become vegan, but I hate vegetables, love meat, and don't have any health problems or moral reasons that I need to switch, then it's not a goal that I'm going to be able to stick to. That doesn't make me weak or lazy, the goal just didn't match my priorities.

Most people are not lazy, they are uninspired. You need goals that match their real priorities so they are internally motivated to achieve them! When you find the right goal, you will know because you will get excited thinking about it, working toward it, and envisioning it. Your goal must be something you'd genuinely, enthusiastically like to see happen. If it doesn't motivate you, that doesn't mean your lazy; it means that you need a new goal that you are passionate about.

Measurable - Don't make your goal "Get fit," make it "Lose 4 pounds of fat by the end of the month." Look for quantifiable numbers and facts. Don't make your goal "Get strong," make it "Work up to doing 20 push ups in a row by the end of the summer." You can't figure out the steps you need to take to reach your goal until you know exactly what you want to achieve.

Purposeful - "If it is important to you, you will find a way. If not, you'll find an excuse." You need a singular focus on completing your goal. If you'd like to exercise more but, more than that, you'd like to sit on the couch and relax, guess which one you're going to do? Your IMPACT goal must have a higher priority in your life than the other, less constructive ways you could spend your time. Otherwise, those other higher priorities are your true goals, and the ones you will actually achieve.

Active - Our IMPACT goal must be one that we can take specific steps to achieve. At the time we create it, we decide on at least 2 or 3 concrete steps we can take to move us closer to that goal. If we want to lose fat, we can start jumping rope for 15 minutes every morning and start having fresh fruit for dessert instead of sweets.

If we want to make our kids a higher priority, we

can start coaching their soccer team, doing art projects with them, or read to them every night. Choose specific actions that you can take which will bring you closer to your IMPACT goal.

Controllable - Our IMPACT goal must be under our control. We can't force our bosses to give us raises, or force our spouses to have better relationships with us. But, we can control the quality of our work, and invest more time and energy building our relationships with the people who matter the most to us.

Time Specific - As Henry Ford said, "You can't build a reputation on what you are going to do." If we decide we'll try to accomplish a goal whenever we get around to it, it will never happen.

We must set a specific date that we want to have achieved our goal by. This date is what motivates us to take action today, instead of always planning on starting tomorrow.

Welcome to the Jungle

Every thought and movement you make comes from split-second electrical impulses in your brain. Whether you do a math problem, order dessert, smile, or lift a weight it's all caused by electrical impulses in your brain.

Star performers start out like everyone else, but, over the course of years of effort, they improve the wiring in their brains. When you exercise, skip dessert or decide to go to sleep early, specific areas of your brain activate in sequence.

Most of the electrical impulses in these sequences die out out along the journey through your brain. If your brain starts out with a signal at 100%, with new tasks, only 10% or 20% of the initial mental signals will come through, most of the signal is lost along the way.

Concentration and practice slowly wraps the thought and movement patterns that you concentrate on in myelin sheathes, which insulate the pathways and keeps the electrical impulse from leaking out along its journey.

It's the difference between trying to stay warm in winter in a t-shirt and trying to stay warm in a thick coat. The insulation doesn't create the energy, but it traps it inside and keeps it from escaping. It means a little bit of focus goes a long way!

Beginners may have virtually no myelin sheathes in areas of the brain used on new things, while experts may have built up multiple layers of myelin insulation. This means the same mental exertion that a beginner puts out will come through in a much greater way for an expert because the physical makeup of their brain has changed and less energy is lost, which leads to more trained thought and action, without as much mental strain.

Babies will strain to take their first steps using all their mental and physical focus, but in time, they can walk around effortlessly without even thinking about it.

An amateur pianist may not be able to make it through "Mary Had a Little Lamb" but an experienced concert pianist can play the complex melodies of Mozart's symphonies.

Think of your mind like an untamed jungle filled with dense trees, vines, and bushes. Getting through it is almost impossible and is slow and exhausting work.

Eventually you make it through, and, when you look back, you notice the path you took through the jungle. You pushed vines aside, and your feet kicked some of the trip hazards out of the way. You can see that your steps made the beginnings of a path for you to follow next time.

Over time, you keep following the same path, and the vines, trees, and bushes will be worn away until you have an easily cross-able dirt road, free of obstructions—you can now run through quickly and easily. This is exactly what happens in your mind every time you take a particular action, whether it is practicing a physical movement or making a specific choice.

You build the myelin sheath in your brain corresponding to that action and clear the pathway for easier and faster travel. The more you focus and force healthy habits and thoughts initially, the faster you will build myelin sheathes and the more effortlessly your new healthy choices will flow.

At first, making any healthy new lifestyle change will feel like you're pushing through a dense physical and emotional jungle, but as you repeat it over time it will become a effortless and automatic!

You Hate to Lose!

We **hate** depriving ourselves of things. If you tell me I can't have a jelly bean I'll suddenly want one, and I don't even like jelly beans! That's okay, we can use our hatred of deprivation to **guarantee** that we achieve our goals.

I am going to share a powerful psychological technique called cognitive reprogramming with you. We are loss averse and get more upset at the prospect of losing something than we get happy about the prospect of getting the same thing. When we focus on what we stand to lose, we react strongly to keep it! So, if we feel like we are depriving ourselves of steak or sweets, we'll just want it that much more.

Therefore, instead of framing situations in terms of what you are depriving yourself of, flip it and focus on what you're getting. You're not missing out on eating Oreos. You're enjoying a nutritious meal that's going to give you the body you want as well as plenty of mental and physical energy.

You're not depriving yourself of chocolate cake, you're ensuring that at your college reunion next month everyone comments on how amazing you look. Focus on what you **would** be depriving yourself of if you indulged.

By eating that ice cream, you would be depriving yourself of showing off your sexy 6 pack abs at the beach this summer. You'd be depriving yourself of how good you'd feel looking in the mirror and loving who you see looking back at you. You'd be depriving yourself of how strong you'd feel controlling your eating, instead of letting your eating control you.

Taking time to visualize your new body and imagining looking in the mirror and seeing the new you is a great way to stay motivated. As Zig Ziglar said, "People often say that motivation doesn't last. Well, neither does bathing - that's why we recommend it daily."

When you remind yourself what you'd be missing out on if you ate badly, it becomes **much** easier to stay disciplined. Sacrifice is giving up something good for something better. Always focus on "What you're choosing, not what you're losing."

"Nothing tastes as good as looking good feels." - Anthony Robbins

#7 How to Empty Your Fat Bank

"To accomplish great things, we must not only act, but also dream; not only plan, but also believe." - Anatole France

Refresh & Review

Lets do a quick review of the major Empty Your Fat Bank concepts we've covered:

Your body wants to prepare itself to survive a long period of starvation by lowering the amount of calories it requires to function, so it's fat stores will last it long enough to find it's next meal. It does this by producing a hormone called cortisol that slows down your calorie burning.

By following a few basic rules, you can kill your cortisol levels, keep your body out of starvation mode, and keep your metabolism speeding along like a fat-burning furnace.

Live Like a Millionaire!

What if you got a check for 1 million dollars every day for the rest of your life? I doubt you'd worry much about how much you had in the bank!

The only way to convince your body that you genuinely don't need fat stores is to feed it healthy snacks every few hours and convince it that there are no threats to future access to a food supply, to avoid setting off your cortisol emergency trip wires. This is the one and only situation in which you can easily, quickly and continuously shed fat.

After all, if your body is getting fed regularly, and it will continue to, why does it need to keep stored calories around? Here is a list of what we've discussed up to this point, and quick easy steps you can take to avoid tripping your cortisol wires and keep your Fat Bank open for constant withdrawals.

Chapter #2 Food & You: How to Make Fat Bank Deposits

Never skip breakfast, always eat something as soon

as you wake up. Eat small meals regularly every 3-4 hours. Avoid refined sugar and emphasize foods that break down slowly like fruits, vegetables, lean proteins, and foods high in fiber. If you are going to eat sugar, try to have it at breakfast, right before a workout or right after a workout, the 3 times it is least likely to be stored.

Chapter #3 Exercise & You: How to Make Fat Bank Withdrawals

You don't need to workout for hours a day to lose fat or gain muscle. 30-60 minutes, 3-4 times a week is plenty. More time than that can actually stop you from building muscle or burning fat. Building muscle is the best permanent weight control method to keep fat off long term, because maintaining muscle will use up calories that would otherwise be stored as fat.

You'll always get the most out of workouts if you get a small snack or sports drink before you exercise so you have plenty of energy to really push yourself. If you are having a hard time motivating yourself to exercise, start hitting the gym with a friend, experiment with new sports and exercise classes, and use your favorite foods as rewards that you can only have if you workout.

Chapter #4 Sleep & You: How to Open Your Fat Bank Vault

Getting enough sleep is the single most important thing you can do to to open you Fat Bank vault. If you easily lose track of time, try setting a bedtime alarm to remind you when you should start getting ready for bed. This will ensure that you get your full

8 hours and don't get distracted. Try to keep a regular bedtime and waking time everyday to get the most out of your sleep. When you are trying to go to sleep, avoid distractions like action movies, or video games, go for a boring book to knock you out. Avoid caffeine, sugar, and other stimulants before bed. If you have things on your mind keeping you up, take a few minutes and write them down. This will clear your head and let you take care of them in the morning. Exercising earlier in the day will help tire you out physically, so you can go to sleep more easily at night.

Chapter #5 Stress & You: How to Keep Your Fat Bank Vault Open

All of us feel overworked and over-scheduled with more to do than is realistically possible. That is the permanent state of modern life, and the only way to strive in our environment is to accept that there will always be much more to do, than can ever be done.

When we come to terms with this fact and stop feeling like we could, or should, do everything, we can finally start to pick our battles. By saying no to more work and tasks that drain us of our energy, we have more time to focus on our most important goals. We are completely free to give our undivided focus to our top priorities, instead of being distracted by things that aren't as important to us.

By taking a few moments each morning to envision how we will make that day our masterpiece, we can set goals that will helps us get the most from our days. Set aside specific goals, some sacred you time, and you will be shocked how much better you feel and how much more you accomplish with your time.

Chapter #6 Food & You:

How to Automate Your Fat Bank Withdrawals

We are built to grow. What we can do tomorrow isn't defined by what we can do today. You may not be able to do 20 pushups right now, but with exercise and healthy meals, you can quickly work up to it. Likewise, today you may not have the discipline to drastically change your routine, and adopt a completely new lifestyle. But if you take baby steps in the right direction, you will build your confidence and your momentum.

You will make mistakes along the way, but every time you say no to that indulgent desert and yes to that workout will make it easier, until it becomes completely effortless.

But how do you break through your initial inertia and the comfort of your old habits? You need to set specific targets, and build a goal system to help you achieve them. This system will push and support your success, even when you wouldn't feel motivated by yourself. This will carry you through the hardest parts of the adjustment, until your new lifestyle becomes a comfortable self-sustainable routine that is familiar and friendly to you.

#8 Conclusion

"Today is a new day." - Chicken Little

"Now this is not the end. It is not even the beginning of the end. But it is, perhaps, the end of the beginning." - Winston Churchill

New Response Ability

You now have a new responsibility. Well, actually not a responsibility, but a **response ability**.

Before you read this, when it came to losing fat, you didn't know the secrets that you needed to change your body. No one ever gave you the guidance or knowledge you needed to Empty Your Fat Bank.

A 4 year old can't perform open heart surgery, even if he or she genuinely wants to help the patient. If someone is mugged in a nearby city, even if I would like to intervene and help, I am in another city and thus cannot be held responsible. Likewise, even if you had the best intent and made a Herculean effort, before you read this book, you could not change your body because you did not have the knowledge you needed.

But today, after learning the secrets and strategies to Empty Your Fat Bank, you have the ability to effectively respond to your desire to lose fat.

You don't lose or gain fat magically. It's all a result of the direct cause and effect of your actions. After reading this book, you know exactly what to do to get the results you want. From this day forward, you are now equipped with a "Response Ability." You are now able to respond to your desire to improve your body and your life!

"Knowing is not enough, we must apply. Willing is not enough; we must do." - Johann von Goethe

Proven Principles

I hold a degree in Psychology, and I have been certified as sports nutritionist and National Council on Strength and Fitness Personal Trainer. Empty Your Fat Bank is the condensed secrets I've learned in my last decade of continuous research. These guiding principles and lifestyle changes have already helped many others empty their Fat Bank, and I can promise that these secrets will also work for you. Remember when I said I used to weigh over 250 pounds? Today, I've lost over 100 pounds of fat and gained over 40 pounds of muscle. That dramatic transformation has taken place solely because I've applied the exact principles that I've shared in these pages.

If I knew when I was starting out what I know now —the information I'm giving you—I could have made twice the progress with half the time and effort. Armed with this powerful knowledge, you can rapidly completely transform the way that you look and feel!

Fitness is not something you are born with. Fitness is not a destination anyone can reach. We can all be a little stronger, or run a mile a little faster. Fitness is a constant journey that we can all make progress on. Start small with short and long-term goals. Don't try to lose 10 pounds in 10 days because your body will think it's starving and slam your Fat Bank vault door shut, putting your fat burning on pause. A healthy goal for most beginners is to lose 1-2 pounds of fat a week with a combination of diet and exercise, and gain 1-2 pounds of muscle a month. You could very reasonably plan to drop 4 pounds by this time next month. If you can do 5 pushups today, try to work up to 10 in 2 weeks.

Whatever your goal is, it has to be something that gets you excited. You need to imagine yourself effortlessly banging out those pushups, fitting into those pants that you haven't been able to wear for years, or looking down at your new toned stomach and smiling. If the goal doesn't inspire you to act, it's not the right goal for you. You need to pick other goals until you find the one that motivates you. That said, try to be realistic, and err on the side of safety. I'd much rather aim a little low and dramatically exceed my goal (tried to lose 1 pound and lost 2) instead of being disappointed that I didn't achieve my goal (tried to lose 20 pounds and lost 2). The difference between victory and defeat is not determined only by what you achieved, but by how much progress you made towards your chosen goal. So choose a careful balance between a goal that is small enough for you to confidently achieve it, but big enough to motivate and inspire you.

Continue your journey into the world of fitness. You now know everything that you need to successfully manage your Fat Bank. You know how to make deposits, withdrawals, open the vault, and keep it open. Now, open your Fat Bank vault, and empty it for good! You have a sexy body ready to show off, you just need to use these secrets and set your body free from the fat. You can do it, just remember to always make your goal, "Progress, not perfection."

If you've found the methods I've taught to be valuable, please share them with others. Good luck, I wish you every success in training and in life.

- Barry Rabkin